The Healing Patch Cookbook

*A gentle transition from cooked to raw foods,
with a joyful taste of wit*

Written by **Julie Cara Hoffenberg**
with **Sarah Woodward**

Healing Patch Publishing
Ojai, CA

Published by Healing Patch Publishing
Ojai, CA 93023

www.rawhealingpatch.com

ISBN: 978-0-578-02813-2

Written by Julie Hoffenberg with Sarah Woodward

Design and Layout by Sarah Woodward

Edited by   Deborah Sindon
                Heather Woodward
                Vincente E. Woodward

Put a child in a room with a lamb and a banana. Note which one he plays with and which one he eats.

- Dr. Douglas N. Graham from <u>The 80/10/10 Diet</u>

DEDICATIONS & ACKNOWLEDGEMENTS

From Sarah:

Ophena – You always challenge me in the kitchen!

Mom - Thank you for teaching me the meaning of flavor; Sicilian style.

Dad – The importance of freshly picked herbs came from you.

Lisa – When I was inspired to cook, you always bought the ingredients.

Dave – You were the first to acknowledge my garlic-dicing abilities so we could make your greasy taco delights!

I would like to thank my grandmothers and great grandmothers for always creating food preparation jobs for the children. Some of my fondest memories include eavesdropping on the grandmothers, while pulling the tips off of green beans. I have learned that the most interesting stories are told in the kitchen.

From Julie:

Mom – You were always making something delicious and cooking 'round the clock. Thank you for leaving deseeded bowls of watermelon and fresh fruit on the counter for the kids. This influenced my ability to come back to the healthy way of life that I now live!

Dad – Or shall I call you "the machine?" Ha ha! Your physical abilities keep me inspired and I dream of the day we will bike ride across the U.S. together! I will like that "rill well."

Grandma Anne - You always had "a 'lil sum-m" ready for me to snack on. Thank you for keeping Nona's recipes alive (and our family history). You are very important to me. Let's grab a crab. xoxoxo

Jon – Laughter keeps me as healthy as any food I could eat. Thank you. "Gobble gobble gobble! I have a brisket prepared for you to take home on the plane. May I help you? How may I help you?"

My female relatives – You are, and were, ALWAYS the cooks. Like Nona said, "Add some salt till it's nice." Bubbe Miriam always appreciated a midnight French fry with me after work even though Arby's didn't add enough "goddamn salt!"

CONTENTS

CONTENTS

Sauces / Dressings

Entrees

Desserts

Appendix

INTRODUCTION

Another raw food book?! Why on earth are we writing the next book on a currently saturated subject? These are the questions we ask ourselves as we delve into this project. Sarah and I, Julie, your writer and M.C. of the fabulous Healing Patch duo, tend to be less extreme than many of the folks out there. We are ever-researching, ever-experimenting, and ever-evolving gals who believe the often harsh and abrasive approach to raw food is not the best choice for everyone.

Okay, peeps (or peep, if there happens to be just one set of eyes reading this), here is the deal: THERE ARE **MANY** VALUABLE, VALID, AND HEALTHY WAYS TO LIVE A VEGETARIAN/RAW FOOD LIFESTYLE. We have researched a great deal on the topic of raw food, nutrition, and health. Most books are loaded with wonderful information and recommendations, backed up with research. See our list in the back of this book for suggested reading. We do not pretend to be doctors or queens of the health world, but we do know that the transition to raw food is different for everyone.

There are a select few who can be sloppily eating a set of spare ribs with a plastic bib tied around their necks one day...and suddenly wake up the next morning with a plate of kale and a cup of homemade sprouted nut mylk! For those of you who can be this hardcore, we ask of our readers, "Can we get an amen?!"

To which y'all should reply, "Oh hells yes! Amen, sistas and bruthas!"

Holy Guacamole! (See our recipe. Not only is this my favorite phrase, it also happens to be my favorite dip.) We respect, honor, and tremble in the wake of such almighty vessels who take the overnight approach.

I have had brief moments of the intense approach above. During cleanses, I am intense. I generally choose times such as the winter holidays for cleansing. One may find me seated at a family dinner with a quart of juice as everyone else hogs down on a plethora of fatty meaty goodness. I must tell you, I love the torture!

Sarah tends to be a bit less intense than me in this regard. As we near the end of a month-long cleanse, she'll say, "Dude, I'm done. Let me know when you're ready. It's time to eat."

She brings some balance to my often anal retentive, torturous approach!

Some of you reading will decide to climb uphill until you reach the threshold of raw food. Others will slowly and tentatively take one new step up a gentle slope and may never reach a total raw food lifestyle. The beauty of these two options is that each approach will bring you forward.

Sarah and I are only two people, choosing our own routes. The right to choose your process is not in our hands; you hold all of the power.

Transitioning from cooked food to vegetarian, or possibly raw, is something that we wish to be as smooth as possible for you. What place do we have in relation to your raw food/vegetarian transition? That is for you to decide.

Perhaps we are just another book on your long list that gives you a small nudge to get going. Maybe we are the spark that starts a completely new life full of fiery health. At the bare minimum, we can begin by sharing a bit of our backgrounds and experience to help you along your way.

WHO THE HECK ARE WE?

Sarah and I make up The Healing Patch Raw Cuisine. We are both a dream and a reality. Our ultimate vision is to create a place of healing, complete with a raw food café, bookstore, meditation space, and garden.

It is rather shocking to find so many wonderful health food stores that sell books, and yet there is nowhere to read! We believe education should be free. If customers would like to learn about their health and educate themselves before purchasing food or supplements, they should have a nice comfy chair to do their research! Perhaps some healing music and the trickle of a nearby fountain may help them focus and raise their vibration. Sarah and I dream of the finest store/café and place of healing, and hope to manifest it when the time is right.

Fortunately, The Healing Patch is not only a dream, but a reality we are living every day! You are holding the first physical "baby" birthed from the company. We have a few other projects going, such as free YouTube health videos, organic seeds for sale, and a health newsletter. You can find these on our website at www.rawhealingpatch.com.

The first bullet point on our list of "to dos" is to help people make the choice to get healthier. We feel writing is the best way to accomplish this quickly and without pressuring people.

There is something sacred about choosing which book to read next. Have you ever noticed that people generally pull a book from the shelf, hold it, fan the pages, and then move on to the next book until it "feels right"? Obviously, they are not reading the book as they go through this ritual. They are, rather, sensing the energy of the book and deciding if it matches their need in the moment. This is how we wish to reach people!

Right now, as I write, I am infusing this book with loving and healing energies. I intend to draw people to this book that need information, laughter, and recipes to embark upon a CHOSEN life of health. Sarah and I *know* that this is not the only raw food book on the planet, but we do know that, for all who choose it, it is perfect.

A BLESSING FOR YOUR HEALTH, LAUGHTER AND HAPPINESS

Sarah and I CHOOSE a healthier way of life than the one we previously lived. Our before-and-after photos speak for themselves. (I just threw away my envelope of "Fat Girl Photos" I saved for the book. Hallelujah!)

Before

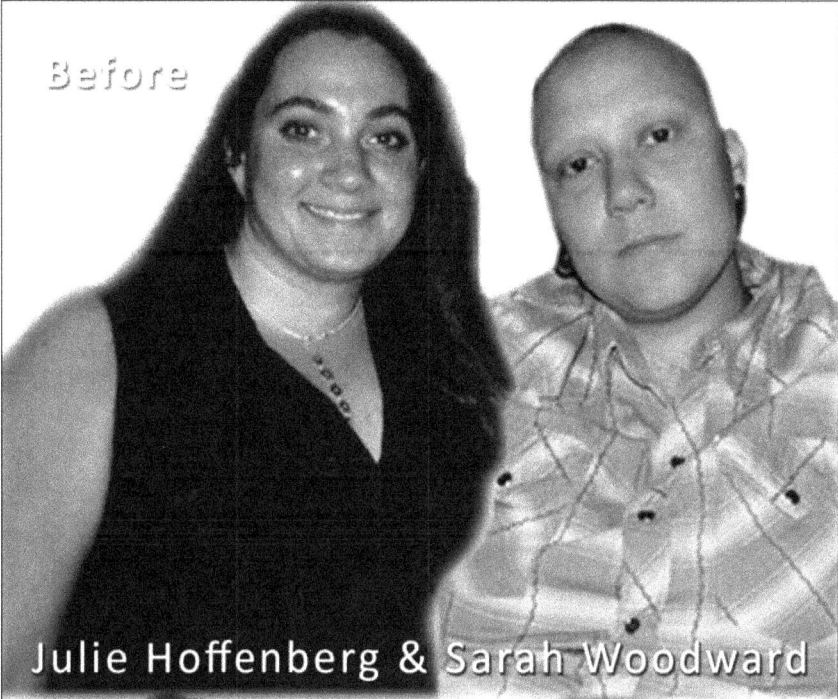

Julie Hoffenberg & Sarah Woodward

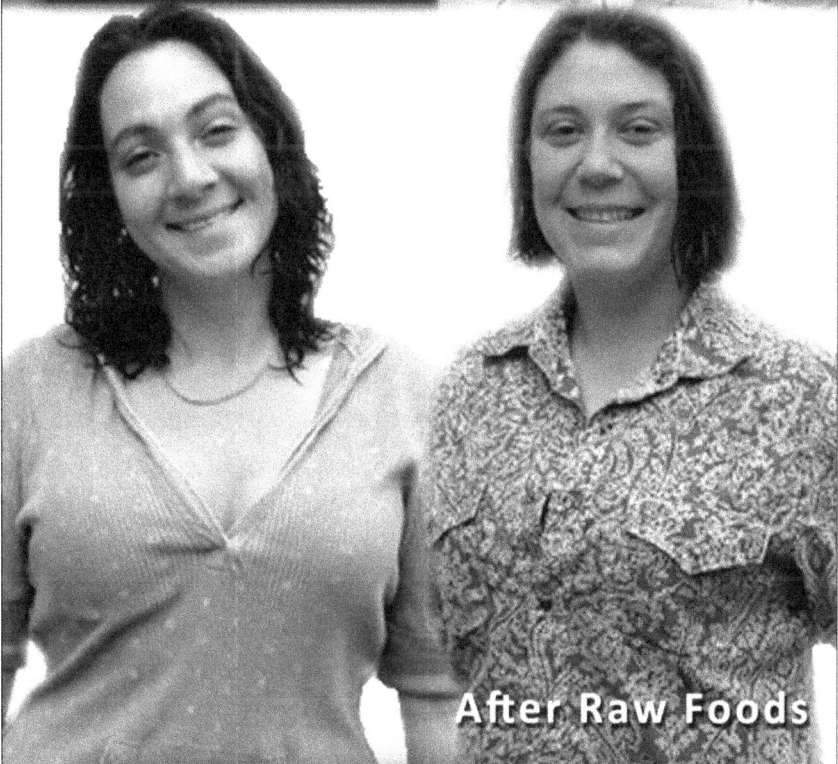

After Raw Foods

As you can see, Sarah was enduring the ever-graceful-and-sexy experience of chemotherapy. She is now healthfully and happily thriving after late stage three ovarian cancer. I have absolutely NO concept or understanding of anything she lived through, as I met her about a year after the chemo treatments. The photos of Sarah during this time period are like the glowing spots I see when I close my eyes tightly. No matter how hard I try, I cannot focus on one spot to make it last. When I glance at the glamorous-baldy-cancer photos, it's also as if they appear and disappear. Sarah is now of completely different energy, and therefore the photos do not register for more than a brief moment.

How did Sarah get into raw foods? She met my crazy health-nut self! When we met, she was a carnivore who ate a basically healthy cooked diet with occasional junk food days.

I was nearly vegan and was beginning to do less and less raw fruits and vegetables in honor of potato chips. If you browse my lovely before picture, you will see that a cooked vegetarian diet did nothing for my beautiful acne, rosacea, or voluptuous figure. Now don't get me wrong, I love me some curves; but they were not healthy curves at that point! They were the full road-size curves they warn you about while driving. I now believe there is a correlation between the warning of imminent danger on the road and the potential danger of an overly abundant toosh! Perhaps our doctors should give US a warning: Caution - Curves Ahead May Lead to Disease.

My seven or so years of experience in the natural health field provided plenty of training, reading, and researching. I was not, however, practicing a whole lot of what I had researched. A feeling of being stuck came over me, which was like standing alone in quicksand. I just could not move anymore (figuratively and physically). What scared me most is that I was not vastly overweight, yet I felt so horrible. This feeling created the momentum to choose a different path. It had been my previous assumption that extremely obese people got stuck in life. Ding dong, I was wrong!

A gentleman working for me was a raw foodist and had the most gorgeous skin I had ever seen. He had energy that was abundant; the kind of energy that I had been dreaming of. I did a cleanse he recommended, which happened to contain only live foods, and my life was never the same. While I continued to ping pong around with my diet, it was the memory of how fantastic I felt during those days of cleansing that propelled me forward.

Suddenly, I was reading all I could on the topic of vegetarian and raw foods. I quit my crap-ass (technical term) job, moved to California, continued researching, and met Sarah. We started making more and more raw meals.

One evening, Sarah and I began reading David Wolfe's phenomenal book, Eating for Beauty. Sarah's mom was visiting and we sat on the couch reading the book out loud together as her mom listened and questioned. I could just imagine it must have looked like I was trying to indoctrinate Sarah into some sort of cult or madness! Now her mom enjoys our recipes (begs for them) and shortly after reading the book Sarah sent me a text message that said she is hanging up her pots. Time to eat raw!

Here we are. Reading more, questioning constantly.

Chapter One will go into the various paths to raw food we researched and give you some guidance as to what you may gravitate towards. We are not yet "100% raw". Family food seems to be the main addiction that we pounce on like wild cats on mice! I still battle a serious love of cheese, while meat is not so much of an issue. The footage of what happens on farms to kill our meat disgusts me in every way, so I can generally steer myself away from it. But cheese, glorious cheese, is such a difficult thing to bury forever. If you stuck me on an island alone with all the fresh fruit in the world and perfect health; I would still say (to myself, obviously), "Where can a girl get a nice slab of brie around here?"

Cripes! It's bad. But I am strong.

Sarah and I are gentle and loving with ourselves. We are not the people out there starting diets on Monday and punishing ourselves for not being perfect. In fact, on the days we eat less than healthy, we laugh at ourselves as we waddle off to bed farting. As you can see, we are also honest.

Our house is always full of fresh, organic fruit and vegetables. We do not purchase refined foods and keep them in our cabinets at home. Eating out with friends and family is generally the time we splurge. Each time we splurge, however, we become more sensitive to the unhealthy foods. Therefore, these rendezvous with cooked food tend to occur less and less.

We would like you to be gentle and loving with yourself as well. This is why we have included a couple of divine cooked food recipes (that are still vegetarian). If some of you are eating meat and dairy still, try the cooked recipes first and then move on to the raw stuff. If you goof up, no worries! Everyone goofs up. (Unless you are the hardcore kale and nut mylk person mentioned at the beginning of the introduction.) We have learned that goofing up is just that; it does not change your next moment.

You have simply given yourself the opportunity to make a better choice.

So keep reading, invite some friends over, and make your first delicious Healing Patch treat!

PATH – ological
PATH – alicious
PATH – of least resistance

"Where do I begin on the raw path?" This is one of the most important questions you can ask yourself.

There are too many books to possibly read, too many articles to look up, and too many experts claiming to know the truth. But you must start somewhere on the road of education.

We recommend you get every bit of information you can, within the hours you have during your hectic lives. Create an hour before bed or set your alarm for an hour earlier in the morning to read raw food, vegetarian, and health books. These books will be your guiding lights that will lead you to shore.

There is no one, specific way, to be a vegetarian. Many leaders in the arena will have you believe there is one ultimate path and should you not choose it, you will never be healthy. If anyone creates this sort of attitude, find a new preacher! We think it is great when experts give solid research to support their view and tips to be healthy on their program. But when they start giving us reasons why their way is the ONLY way, and all other ways lead to demise, a caution flag arises.

First of all, we are all human. No one is the ONE, TRUE, PERFECT, EXCLUSIVE channel for all godly information. (Except, of course, our friend Deborah, who we go to for random feedback and information on EVERYTHING...chuckle chuckle.) Every time science and research comes up with "the proven truth", things change. Therefore, Sarah and I allow for the possibility that all of the experts have something we may learn. They all have a special way of viewing health and healing. It is our recommendation that you drink in each tasty sip the experts give you, decide if it tastes right and is hydrating, then move on to the next drink for a new set of minerals and nourishment.

If we have learned anything, it is that those who create a feeling of fear are not experts. A glass of lemonade must contain lemons. Similarly, a fear-mongering expert must also be full of fear, for we may only pour out the energy we hold within ourselves.

"What do these health gurus fear," you ask?

There is the potential fear you will not continue to buy their books, products, or whatever else they may be selling. These are the folks who tell you that you may die early if you do not follow their exact program. Luckily, there are very few of these dogma-spewing people in the health world; but there are a few, so heads up!

When we find experts who give the option of their path, explain that other paths may not be perfect, but you may stay fairly healthy on them, we know they are not full of fear. There are people all over the planet living VASTLY different lives and eating NOTHING like one another. *Many* of these groups are vibrantly healthy. If there was only one path that would sustain a lifetime of health, this would not be the case.

We appreciate the grace of gentle, intelligent experts and authors. One of which is John Robbins. He wrote the following quote in his book, The Food Revolution. It typifies the qualities an expert should have; the openness to give us the research and explanations, and the ability to trust that there are exceptions to the rule (without allowing it to attack their ego).

I do not believe that, in this society, we can become fully compassionate, conscious beings without deeply questioning the food we eat. But that does not mean any of us are to blame for the illnesses we might experience. I'm talking about greater self-responsibility here, not greater guilt. None of us should ever be made to feel a failure for becoming sick, or for failing to cure ourselves. None of us should ever be made to feel that we are letting ourselves or anyone else down if we become ill. Eating healthfully raises your odds of being well. It greatly reduces your risk of many diseases, and it opens the door to experiencing new levels of joy and passion and purpose in your body. But it cannot guarantee that you won't become ill.

The research undeniably shows that vegetarian and low meat diets create lives with less disease, but there are numerous paths to take and many of them will keep you healthy. For now, we will keep researching and then pass forward the info! The list of books we have provided at the back of the book is a small slice of the whole pie. Start there and add your own new treasures. In the meantime, we will explain some of the various paths people choose so that you may begin to take that first step in a way that makes sense for you.

PATH-ological

While there are many meanings for the word "pathological," I use this term to refer to those people who become pathological liars. Many people embarking on a raw food diet jump in so quickly without any understanding of the lifestyle, that they are driven by their addictions to hide the truth of what they are eating.

If you have a refrigerator filled with avocadoes, strawberries, and lettuce and find yourself sitting in a fast food parking lot on your way home from work, you may be taking the PATH-ological route! Perhaps your friends take you out to eat and you kindly smile and order a plain side salad with a lemon wedge since you are now such an awesome-lean-machine raw foodist! However, as soon as you leave the parking lot, you are off to Trader Joe's for a few microwavable pizzas, a bag of corn puffs, and some chocolate chip cookies.

There are many people who follow this path. The raw food diet is no different from other diets that people begin, if they have not researched and have no clue about actual health! Therefore, people binge and lie until they understand what the heck they are doing and how to deal with, or prevent, withdrawal.

Guilt is not necessary if you are on the PATH-ological route. Admit this is where you were, and CHOOSE a new experience right now. Make the choice to read more books until you understand how to really go about life as a raw foodist.

Perhaps you do not need to be 100% raw right now. Steam up some veggies with goat cheese melted on top and enjoy a nice bowl of homemade soup as you continue to add more raw foods to your diet.

There is no research we have found that proves cooking food increases its level of nutrition without compromising other benefits of the food. For example, beans may be more digestible cooked, as some of the enzyme-inhibitors have been rinsed and cooked away; but most of the vitamins, antioxidants, and enzymes have been killed in the process. That is why we stick with mostly raw.

Sarah and I tend to live a predominantly raw food lifestyle and never have any problems going back to raw foods if we eat a bit of cooked food. We shop our farmer's market EVERY week, which keeps our house full of fresh, ripe food. Raw food is not something we force ourselves into because we know it's healthier; it is cuisine that we have come to love and feel best on.

If you get to this point, it is just no big deal anymore to eat raw food. You may have a night where the tantalizing, beckoning call of pizza wafts through your nostrils, so you decide to indulge yourself. Despite the constipation from the cheese, the fatigue from the wheat, and the water retention from the salt (how sexy); do not take the PATH-ological route! There is no need to beat yourself up, lie to others (and yourself), and feel like a failure. If you are in the pattern of eating and loving a very high ratio of raw to cooked food, the whole experience will be rather funny! You will easily wake up the next day, grab some greens or a smoothie, and move on with life.

We do not recommend you do the above pizza binge often. It just happens to be a very common occurrence and we believe there is a better path than the lies. When, and if, you get to the point of being 100% raw vegan without reservation, the thought of pizza is not an issue. You are incredible and can just skip right on to Chapter 2, as you are obviously not battling the "Which path do I take?" issue.

Allow me to move on to the next path of choice. Giddy-up, people! Are you still with me?

PATH-alicious

Yet another fork in the road shows up with the name of PATH-alicious. This seems to be the path most often chosen, or happened upon, by newly born raw foodists. I traveled this path for quite some time and sometimes still do. This is what it sounds like. You eat anything and everything that is delicious to your taste buds (but it must be raw/vegetarian).

Oh, sweet Sally! (No, I have no idea who Sally is either.) Am I saying that you can sit down with a jar of coconut butter and a spoon until it is but a memory? Am I saying that you can eat a dressing-drenched raw salad complete with three avocadoes and a bottle of raw olives? Am I saying that you can make a dessert recipe from this book and ravenously truck through the entire thing?

Yes, yes, and yes!

Have I confused thee? Let me explain. When people begin a raw food lifestyle and no longer eat much (or any) meat, dairy, or refined food, they tend to be very hungry. VERY hungry. VERY VERY hungry. Especially when they try to live off of a salad and an apple for the day! This is just pure madness. Your body needs food; plenty of it. The stereotypical image of a twig-like, earth-loving vegetarian/raw foodist is not the norm. Most of us do not live solely off of flimsy amounts of calories that typically come from dark leafy greens and tofu! Many raw foods are very rich and full of dense calories from fat. These are the foods that tend to be delicious when we first go raw. This is where I coined the term PATH-alicious.

Delicious food is what you should enjoy when you are transitioning into your vegetarian/raw food way of life. Because your body was so used to eating refined carbohydrates and fats (which are LOADED with calories), most people can get away with eating huge portions of dense and delicious raw foods, without gaining weight. They also digest food much easier, due to the high enzyme content, which prevents the food from storing up in places like the thighs and booty! I know someone who really did eat a whole jar of coconut butter! And this person kept on losing weight, feeling phenomenal, and eventually mellowed out on the coconut snacks.

I must note that I am not encouraging the practice of gorging yourself on your favorite raw food staples. It must be stated that the initial path of choosing delicious foods can help you get through cravings and withdrawal from addictive cooked foods.

Would we rather you ate a whole raw chocolate mousse dessert, or a pint of Ben and Jerry's chocolate ice-cream? The answer is always the raw food. It will have no refined sugar, no dairy, and will be full of antioxidants and enzymes! Taking the PATH-alicious trail will often keep you heading in the direction you want to go. This option beats jumping off the path and swan diving into a large order of buffalo wings with a quart of ranch for dipping!

Do not worry, my friends. You will not eternally eat forklifts full of raw food. The body slowly tires of huge portions and will not want rich, fatty foods twenty four hours a day. Initially, these large portions may be the pattern, and it is our job to warn you that this is perfectly normal.

We think you are doing a great job if you are on the PATH-alicious route, for you will eventually move right into the next phase. You can also skip this path altogether and choose the following one.

PATH-of Least Resistance

Zippety-doo-dah! We love the PATH-of least resistance! This gentle path leads you to a very intuitive approach, based on the old-time notion that the things we resist seem to come toward us with more and more strength.

Lying to you will do no good. It would be a complete lie to tell you that transitioning into raw food will be perfectly easy and you will have no moments of resisting temptation. We are more than open to, and respectful of, the select few who had an awakening, became raw foodists overnight, and immediately were sickened by the thought of dead food in any form.

I, for one, did not have this instant repulsion to all things unhealthy. Neither did Sarah. We crave things. We resist things. We have moments of self-talk that say, "Get your fingers out of the French fry container and into a bag of organic grapes!"

Choosing the path of least resistance just means listening closely to what your body needs. You must also research and consider what path seems achievable for you and your lifestyle. The path that would create the most resistance, based on the way you live, should be passed over for a choice that grooves with the way you live. For example, there are some vastly different philosophies and approaches to living a raw lifestyle that do not suit everyone's reality or need, but certainly suit some.

David Wolfe is a great example of someone who has a very clear view of how to live raw. (See our suggested reading list.) He is a huge supporter of superfoods, which are concentrated, dense foods full of vitamins, minerals, and anti-oxidants. Raw cacao, spirulina, maca, and goji berries are just a few of the superfoods he advocates. Fat content is not so much of an issue with Wolfe's approach. He does not preach any sort of calorie counting or restrictive practices. Sarah and I tend to view his approach as one that is relatively laid back. He just seems to want people to live a healthier, rawer existence through the use of enzyme rich foods, as well as superfoods. This simplicity, paired with his depth of knowledge regarding superfoods and raw life, convinces us that this path is one we can certainly use to educate ourselves. Eating foods like raw cacao, avocadoes, and goji berries, thus far, has been both satisfying and good on our bodies. How do we know this? By experimenting and observing how we feel while eating these foods. We feel great and stay healthy while eating these items, as well as others Wolfe recommends.

In reality, our cravings sneak up every now and then. Part of what we have researched explains that cravings are addictions. Other materials we have read explain that the cravings are a result of the wrong raw food choices. These poor choices lead to deficiencies in the body, which in turn lead to cravings.

The 80/10/10 Diet by Dr. Douglas N. Graham gave us wonderful insight as to why certain cravings happen. Graham is strictly opposed to raw cacao and other superfoods, as well as high fat intake. His book was the exact opposite approach to raw food when comparing it to David Wolfe's books. On the 80/10/10 program, you would be eating 80% carbohydrates predominantly from sweet fruit and some greens. The other 20% would come from small amounts of fat and protein from nuts, seeds, and fattier fruits.

While we examined both views, as well as many in between, we find little morsels to be gained from both approaches. There is no definite path (yet) that we strictly adhere to except the path of least resistance. At this point, living off of mostly salads while practicing calorie restriction, is not a place that feels balanced. Our minds and bodies immediately want to resist this approach, although we read and appreciate the science behind calorie restriction.

Experts claim that as we slowly begin to eat less, we age slower. This is because all of our energy (life force) is drained during the digestive process. If we eat less, we reserve more life force, and therefore age more slowly. This path makes my stomach grumble just thinking about it! So it is a path of resistance for now. Perhaps this route will not feel resistant in the future, but for now it does.

Try a few approaches as you are doing your research. Some of you will do/feel better on a diet of rich, satisfying raw food recipes filled with dense food. Others will feel energetic and full of light when they eat whole fruits and vegetables unaltered in any way, but if things feel OVERLY strenuous and resistant, you need to make a change.

As you hold the rope, there should be a small tug on the other end sometimes. If that tug is just a craving here and there, it is no big deal. But if every day feels like there is someone pulling on the other end of the rope with all of their strength until you plummet into the abyss of barbeque and potato salad, choose a new path! You are looking for the PATH-of least resistance. We cannot tell you which one will suit you, we can only give you the information you need to research, and the understanding of what is potentially normal and healthy.

We would like to thank all of the raw food experts out there doing the scientific research, sitting around in lab coats, watching blood samples. This is not our department! We can, however, explain all that we have read and hopefully give our wonderful readers a good sense for many of the different paths people choose when going raw/vegetarian. Should any of you come up with an altogether different path not mentioned here, and you are feeling fantastic, we say, "Own it and share it!"

Now carry on to the next chapter, where we try to figure out what's really up with you and your food (fun, fun)!

Apathy/Abstinence
Makin' Sweet Love
Intention

What sort of relationship have you created with your food? Some of you are grimacing at this question right now! Hang in there, I will be gentle. Don't get all paranoid on me now! I am not here to accuse, but rather to shed light on the dark scary places you wish not to go.

Food relationships are important to analyze. These help us decipher why we have cravings and addictions, amongst other things. I am not talking about taking your food out for a first date and wondering whether you should have your first kiss! I am talking about the energy you hold while eating your food, as well as the perceptions you have about what food means to you.

Raw food is full of life (energy), enzymes, and nutrition! What is the point of eating this food, if you are daydreaming about the twelve things you need to accomplish tomorrow? I recently caught myself eating while watching a movie and realized I had no conscious memory of how wonderful the food tasted. This experience led me to question what sort of relationship(s) I have with my food.

APATHY/ABSTINENCE

Raw foodists just embarking on the lifestyle often become apathetic about what they are eating (if they eat much at all). Because the flavors are so vastly different from the ones they ate on a diet full of processed foods, which are full of chemical stimulants, they sometimes become totally disinterested or apathetic towards food.

An example of this sudden taste apathy may be illustrated further. Consider the experience of a cooked food eater who enjoys steaks doused in A1 sauce with a side of flavored chips (full of MSG), suddenly trying a raw food diet of salads with olive oil and vinegar and some sliced bananas. This is not exactly the same flavor explosion!

Eventually, the flavors in raw food become more and more intense as your taste buds adjust to not being constantly over-stimulated. But it takes some time, and this is why people transitioning to raw food often hit the apathy approach. They figure, "Oh hell, I would rather not eat, than eat tasteless crap like that!"

Some people completely refrain from eating enough calories. Because they are apathetic about the flavors, they stop eating most of everything and reach a point of near abstinence. At which point they get hungry and frustrated, leading them to binge on the cooked foods again! The eating cycle can be vicious.

If you have an apathetic or abstinent relationship with food, it would help to add back a few of the cooked foods. They should not contain any additives, refined sugars, or refined starches. Choose foods that are as close to 100% organic as possible. Adding a few cooked, unrefined foods back to your diet will allow the body to slowly move away from the stimulant and refined base of ingredients present in most store-bought shelf products. As you move away from artificial tastes and toward natural flavors, your taste buds will begin to recognize more and more healthful flavors.

Try doing some natural versions of the toxic meals you used to eat. An example of a natural version would be to make steamed broccoli with fresh lemon juice and Celtic sea salt instead of deli counter potato salad. These deli salads are full of toxic preservatives, sugars, etc.... Maybe a dash of organic parmesan on top of your broccoli would satisfy the taste buds. This whole process is about finding healthier options. Sometimes a cooked option in a more healthful form is perfectly fine versus diving into 100% raw and becoming apathetic and frustrated.

MAKIN' SWEET LOVE

The next relationship with food that I observe everywhere I go, is the relationship in which people seem to make sweet love to their food. I bet you have seen this too! The all-you-can-eat buffets are the best place to watch this happen. Here is the scenario:

Scene 1: There is a gentleman with a belly the size of a large pumpkin approaching the buffet behind you. You can feel him scan the buffet and slide his tray closer to yours to get you to move more quickly through the items. He seems to have seen something that he must have on his plate. You are not certain, but believe it is the macaroni and cheese. Wait a minute! Is the macaroni dancing up the buffet structure as if it was a stripping pole? The way he glances at the saucy noodles makes you think this must be taking place.

He is starting to sweat and you can hear his heart beating fast. Thump-a-thump-a. Or should I say Hub-a-Hub-a?! You have barely finished making your salad at the front of the bar, but Mr. Macaroni wants his noodles pronto!

Scene 2: You watch Mr. Macaroni-lover-man skirt around you, smirking at your slow salad making pace. He then begins to smile as he approaches his new "dish." He dives in, unable to control himself. Miss Macaroni has been such a tease and now she is comin' home to Pa Pa!

You, on the other hand, are still adding the toppings to your salad and have not yet scanned the main course area of the buffet.

Scene 3: Mr. Macaroni happens to be sitting at a table adjacent to yours. There is a light sweat on his forehead, his fingers are tapping the table, and he is rubber-necking for the waiter to take his plate so he may get seconds. You wonder how he can eat any more after slurping down a mountain-sized platter of Miss Macaroni. Phew!

Scene 4: Your salad was most delish and you think a few ounces of the soft serve would be a nice finish to your meal.

As you walk up to the soft serve machine, Mr. Macaroni seems to be dating someone new. Miss Sundae. He is ahead of you in line and as he piles a perfectly sculpted Dairy Queen-like set of soft serve mounds onto his bowl, he begins to softly mumble to himself. You are not sure but it sounds like he is mumbling sweet nothings like, "Oh, baby! I love me some sprinkles!" and "Oooohhhh. Warm fudge. I love it!"

You are about to throw up because you watched a man make virtual sweet love to Miss Sundae. Mr. Macaroni is just minutes away from dripping strawberry sauce all over his nipples and calling it a night!

Scene 5: You no longer think soft serve is necessary. Cut. End of scenario.

Does any part or all of that scene sound familiar? We tend to have a very lustful relationship with food. I must include myself here. I am no saint. I can hear myself moan as I approach the cheese island at Whole Foods!

This makin' sweet love relationship with food is not the healthiest place to be. It becomes borderline obsession. Food is our nourishment. It is not our social, physical, and sensual need. It can enhance all of the above, but is not here to fulfill those purposes/needs.

So what am I ultimately saying? If you relate to your food in such a way that breeds constant craving, dreaming, lusting for, impatience for, or you plan activities around food instead of the activity itself, I think you may be in the makin' sweet love phase! What should you do about this? The next food relationship is your mission, and I will discuss things that may help create a healthy relationship with food.

INTENTION

Intention is the only thing you need to remember when you eat. If you intend to create a healthy meal, full of loving infusions and connection to where the food came from; hallelujah!

How do you begin this intention? Through the act of being conscious.

Most of us remain very unconscious when we eat. How many times a day do you look at your plate and wonder where, geographically, your food came from? How often do you prepare a meal in silence? This means there are no interruptions from television, radio, or family. Where is your mind focused when you make your meals? The mission is to become present and conscious when you prepare and eat your food.

Food obsession can often disappear when you learn to focus on food ONLY when you are in the active mode of harvesting or preparing it. We do not need to be dreaming of cupcakes while we do homework. If you are hungry, get up, make a snack, and then return to what you should be focusing on.

I can polish off a serious bag of potato chips as I drift into a movie. When I sit under a tree on a hike and eat potato chips in silence, I tend to put them away after I feel like I have had enough. Why? I am present while eating. It is my intention to eat what my body is feeling like receiving; not an entire bag of chips to aimlessly eat as my mind is occupied with other distractions.

Why does Mom's (or Dad's) home cookin' always taste best? Why is it that when we make the same recipe, it tastes nothing like Mom's? INTENTION.

Mothers stir in their love. They intend to nourish and feed their children with the food they earned from hard work on the job. Some Mothers had gardens. They grew most of their food and intended it to grow, putting all of their energy and focus into good weather and a bountiful harvest. The energy, intent, and love our parents stir into our food create a special blend of tastes. They cannot be duplicated, because we are not in the same frame of intention when we cook the same food! We are generally in the intent of hoping the recipe turns out right, or we are yelling at the kids and cracking open a beer to get through the evening as we prepare the meal. It is time to be present, peeps!

Intend, right now, to begin (or continue) a healthy relationship with food. No apathy, no makin' love, no obsession; just pure intention to create health and nourish the body. Write your intention on the following lines, stated in your own words, of what you wish to create in your relationship with food.

_____
_____
_____
_____
_____

This is the age for getting back to the earth. Hold the peach you bought at the store and look at the sticker. Where did your peach come from? Your own state? Another state? Another country? Another continent? Did you intend to buy fruit from another continent? Did you wake up the other day and say to yourself, "Gosh, I sure cannot stand the local peaches. I am going to have to find a nice batch imported from Ecuador."

If you did not intend to do that, why did you do it? If it is your intention to eat locally grown produce, hop on it! Intend, and it will come.

Our next chapter discusses how much our relationship with food can change the world for the better, as well as our eating habits.

Get on the bus, Gus! (Or rather on a bike, as this will save pollution, but bus rhymes with Gus.) Next stop is the garden!

Chapter 3: PLANT THE SEEDS

Garden
Plate
Planet

Gotta save that...and plant it. Grow my own paw paw patch!
'Course, by the time I'm fifty, yeah, then I'll have some paw paws
but, um, it's somethin' to look forward to.

-Steve O'Neil (a.k.a. Youtube.com/snakesteve68)

YouTube is a jungle we can lose ourselves in. Every now and then we happen upon a new treasure while watching someone's video. This is what happened when I saw Steve O'Neil's video about hunting for wild paw paw fruits. It was a case of perfect synchronicity. I was dreaming up ideas for this chapter and when he said the above quote, it was like a choir began to sing. The quote represents the whole connection to food we should have, from beginning to end.

GARDEN

Steve harvests wild paw paws in the video and saves the seeds. He is a middle aged man and potentially will not see the first harvest of what he plants. His concern, however, is not whether he will see the full grown paw paws. He is simply connected to the experience of watching the plants grow. He also trusts that these plants will yield fruit for the next generation. Are you looking forward to any seeds you have planted?

Apartment-style living does not lend itself to challenge-free gardening, but I do have a few suggestions. If you have windows, you can create window box planters. If you have a balcony, you can grow grapes along the railing/fence or create herb pots. Many herbs grow well indoors and you can grow them on an empty counter space. Perhaps you can make an altar for your plants on an empty wall near a window! After harvesting some of the herbs, allow the plant to go to seed. Collect the seeds for your children, family, and friends.

Community gardens offer another place to grow your own food or watch someone else's. You can inquire about adopting your own plot to grow some food, or perhaps volunteer time to work someone else's plot so that you may benefit from the harvest!

Why am I writing about gardening in a vegetarian/raw food cookbook? Gardening has become something most of us are completely disconnected from. How can we intend to create divine relationships with our food when it is drowned in chemicals, grown thousands of miles away from us, we do not harvest it ourselves, and we have no idea what it looks like from seed to plant?

We do not have to grow 100% of our food to be connected to it. Exotic fruits such as young coconuts and dragon fruit from places far off are certainly specialties I enjoy! Buying fruit and vegetables from other lands helps us learn about new tastes and cultures, and puts us in a place of yearning to travel. Sarah and I cannot wait to go to the South Pacific islands to pick our own noni fruit, pineapples, and durian. Discovering the tantalizing taste of tropical fruit once in a while is perfectly valid, but should not be the overriding rule. We should be predominantly harvesting wild and local food.

Humans need to "dig up," so to speak, their love for gardening and connecting to their food. There is a slow silence that happens when we stand in our garden with the hose and nourish each plant. Our minds are generally not racing around about the project we need to finish at work. For some reason the garden tends to reach up, gently touch our heads with its magic wand, and suddenly our attention is on the growth process. We begin to notice the water seeping slowly into the soil. The newest flower on the strawberry plant brings the excitement of a new fruit. Bees sing and buzz around, as we watch them pollinate, essentially creating our food for us. This is all a very different experience from jumping in the car, heading to the drive-thru, and ordering a triple stack burger with a soda and side of fries. It is even vastly different from going to the store and getting some organic veggies. Allow me to explain why.

We live in California, where a great deal of agriculture takes place. Cherries, peaches, avocadoes, apricots, oranges, lemons and many other produce items grow here. For some reason, I can walk into the grocery store, pick up an avocado, and the label will read "Mexico" or "Peru." My cherries will sit next to a sign proudly declaring they are from Washington. The oranges will often be from Florida. What the hell is going on here?

People are doing two things. First, they are demanding and purchasing out-of-season fruit. For example, when California is out of avocadoes for the season, we demand they be grown elsewhere and shipped here.

Second, we are not growing our own food. We are relying on someone else to do ALL of it for us. If we all had backyard farms, we would eat what seasonally grew. Yes, I do realize not everyone has a yard and believe we should take care of our community members who do not. Also, the local produce manager would not have to hear everyone complain about how last week there were peaches, now they are gone, and could he/she please find some more?

We are grateful for our local organic markets, for we are blessed to have a couple of them that sell mostly locally grown, organic, and in-season produce. But they do not exclusively sell these.

I am conscious about the fact that I buy a head of garlic here and there, which tends to ship in from hundreds of miles away. This creates the demand for garlic year round, which in turn pressures stores to carry it consistently. I am also aware that I can grow all of my own garlic in pots very easily, harvest it, and then refrigerate it to use throughout the year, or pickle it. This awareness brings me to a place where I can now change the connection with my food. I can choose to be more connected with the growth of my own garlic and thereby reduce the support of off-season buying.

Your challenge is to find one or two items to start with that you can grow. Perhaps it is a lemon tree, so you will have year round lemons. (Many varieties produce fruit year round.) Some of you live in very cold climates, so you can choose some indoor herbs or start designing a summer lettuce bed!

Sarah and I believe that if everyone shifted just a degree or two by planting minimal amounts of food staples, the planet would thank us. New, healthy food relationships would also begin.

PLATE

The next time you sit down to eat a full meal, look at your plate. When I say "look," I mean not only to stare at it, but to drink in every ingredient and decipher where it came from. Some things will have no label on them to distinguish where they originated. Ask yourself a couple of questions:

1. Is my food on this plate organic? If not, what chemicals do I think may have been used to sustain this crop? This may involve research into common cultivation practices of that plant.

2. Have any of these plants been genetically modified? Did they start from seeds owned by Monsanto? (More on this shortly...hold please!)

3. Did any of these plants come from my own town? My own state?

4. Is there meat on my plate? If so, how was it killed and was it treated with hormones during its lifetime?

5. Is there any dairy on my plate? If so, did the cows roam freely or were they destined to a life in a mud pit? (If you have the privilege of traveling through central California, you will see that most cows never touch or see grass. They rather stand in mud, complete with their own feces.) Were these cows treated with hormones?

These questions are just a few that will begin to awaken you to the truth about your food. The answers generally are shocking. Often people find out that most of their food was sprayed, the cows were slaughtered or electrocuted without being sure they died immediately, the dairy is full of growth hormones that make the cows chunk up quickly, and most of the plants come from other countries. The process of answering these questions becomes very uncomfortable. You should begin to get angry and dissatisfied with your findings.

So what next?

Support local farmers. Support organic farmers. Support yourself. Create the vision to buy land. Buy land with your brothers and sisters to make it more affordable, and grow your own food! Buy your own goat, and drink your own hormone-free goat milk. When you purchase seeds or plants, research whether or not they come from a branch of companies that Monsanto owns.

In case you have no clue who is Monsanto, he is the closest thing to Satan I could imagine. That is a pretty strong statement, but his level of power over our lives is unbelievable. He is the master of genetic modification, which is the altering of plant genetics to yield a specific result, without care for health outcomes. Monsanto hybridizes everything he can get his hands on, controls much of the world's seed ownership, and often prevents organic farmers from doing their job.

Organic farmers can no longer compete with Monsanto's super-seed creations or his enormous growing fields. He has driven many organic farmers out of business. Sarah and I encourage you to research Monsanto and his mission. We have only provided you with the tip of the iceberg here, for those of you who have never heard of him.

What's the big deal if we have miles and miles of Monsanto's corn or soy growing? First of all, most of these miles of land used to be organic farms that have since been bought out by Monsanto. Second, nature never creates an environment where one crop grows for miles without any other crop in the area. Lastly, soils become depleted of their rich mineral content when the same crop grows year after year in the same field. This type of farming leads to weak plants, which yields pest attacks. The farmers are forced to use chemicals, herbicides, and pesticides to eliminate the pest issue instead of growing things organically as nature intended.

We become messed up in some psychotic cycle of trying to grow things that would NEVER grow naturally should we let them. We begin to use force to grow our food. I imagine a nice corn stalk crying and yelling, "I cannot grow under these conditions."

I reply, "Too bad, sucker! I just changed your genetics and you have no choice."

Forceful growing is the exact opposite of nature's intention.

PLANET

Let us be conscious of the connection we have with our food. Our thoughts should move from the garden, to the plate we eat off of, to the planet.

Our incredible earth does not wish to be saturated with chemicals. The planet wishes to gift us with the natural growth process placed here since the dawn of time. Forests do not grow miles of pine trees in a row with no other plants in sight. Pine trees of all ages, like grandfathers and seedlings grow. Forests are also full of ferns, flowers, root vegetables, and too many others to list. The nature of our planet is to give us the exact balance of fruits and vegetables, seasonally, that we need.

Look to the planet to show you what your gardens should look like and how to care for your farm animals. As you become directly involved with the growing of your food, the food obsessions, born of convenience, will fall away. We will move from a society of drive-thrus and city-block-sized supermarkets to one of backyard (or front yard) gardens. People will begin to connect again to the sacred process of planting, seeding, and harvesting. By the time the food hits the plate, it will not be some random food, picked too early, from distant lands. Our food will be plant-ripened and drenched in flavor. Our taste buds will come alive, along with our relationship to our food.

Raw food lifestyles are something Sarah and I believe will be as common as the standard American way of eating, if we begin to make this food connection. As people spend time on their farms, they will pick their own food and naturally begin to eat raw and vegetarian. No one will want to head out to the field to kill their cow for dinner (after watching it grow for ten years). Instead, people will pick some grapes and lettuces.

Vegetarian and raw food ways of life are just common sense. If we imagine ourselves with fields of our own animals and orchards, as opposed to grocery stores full of anonymous food, we will intuitively eat as herbivores do. As we harvest our food, we will eat it raw, straight from the plant. It will be so scrumptious, we will barely be able to wait to go home and prepare it. We will be clear channels for all of our creative abilities, and will no longer need to grab a coffee to get us through our horrible day at the office.

Planetary connection is, in our minds, the answer to it all. We should not guilt trip and pressure others into becoming raw foodists. People need education and support. Communities and families need to come together to enable this next transition into locally grown food.

As Sarah's daughter, Ophena, picks arugula flowers from the garden and exclaims, "Look! These are the edible flowers we had at school," I think to myself, "this is the answer."

Ophena's excitement about edible flowers matches that of going to get ice-cream. No one told Ophena to go pick arugula from the garden; she made the connection herself. Ophena chose raw food in the moment because she was actively involved in the garden, to plate, to planet process.

This is our wish for you! We hope you can transition gracefully from cooked, to vegetarian and raw foods, through the connection to your planet.

An intuitive tug inside of you is the best nudge to create a more healthful way of life for yourself. It cannot come from some annoying new raw foodist yapping away in your ear, "Oh my gosh. Like I totally feel so good, and like, I SO want to to get healthy. You should eat only raw foods because they will, like, totally make your whole body vibrate on, like, a whole new level! Seriously!"

The message must come from you.

It will come in the moments you read, and suddenly you are full of chills because the message is so clear.

It will come in the moments you press seeds into the earth and cover them, waiting for the first sign of aliveness!

It will come in the moments you tell your children, "Kids! Come with me down to the garden. We need to decide what we are having for dinner!"

To your gardens.

To your planet.

To your most graceful and healthy path.

Here are our recipes. Infuse them with love and connection to nature. Enjoy! We bless them with thanks and love!

-Julie and Sarah xoxo

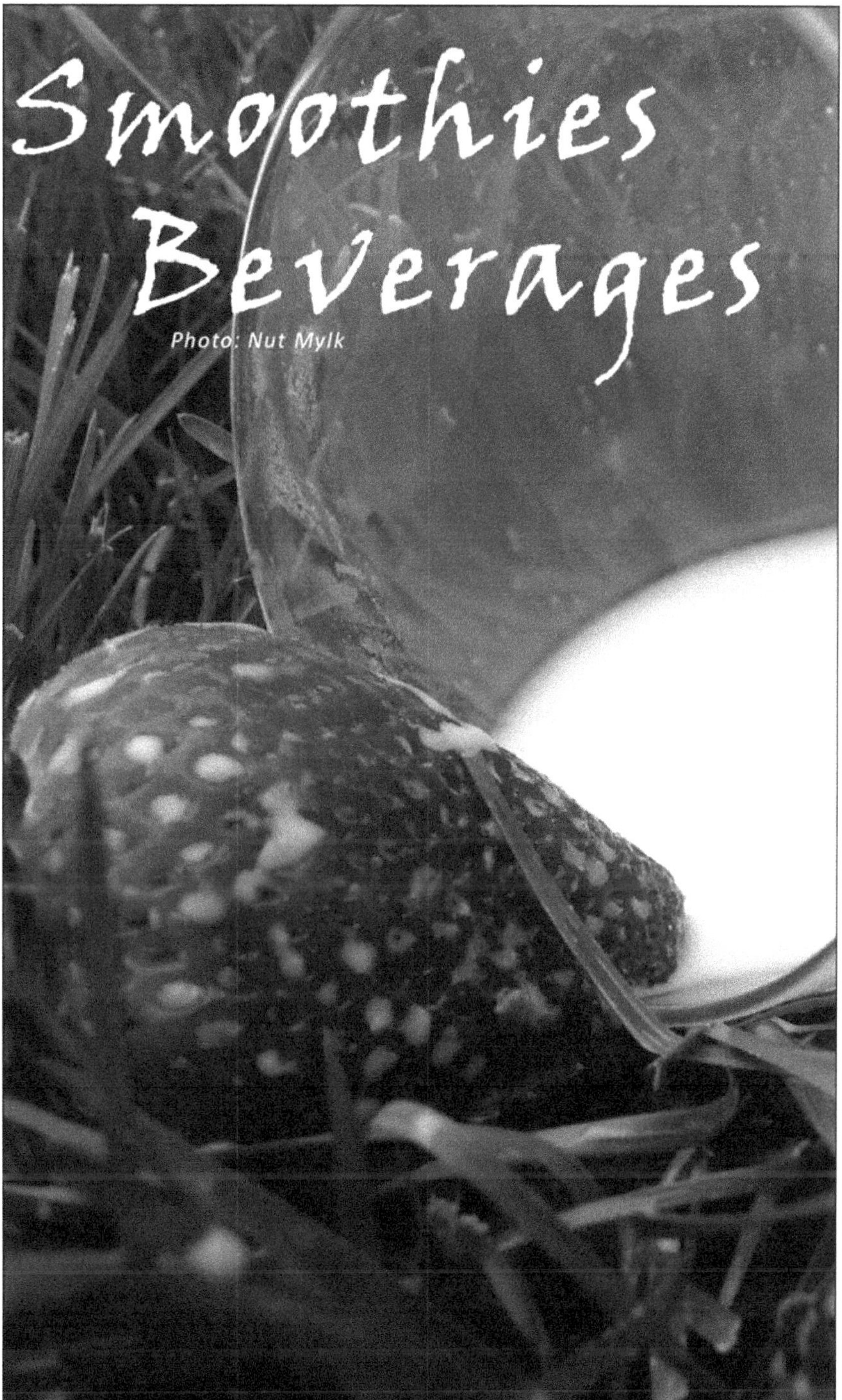

Smoothies
Beverages

Photo: Nut Mylk

PAPAYA COCONUT WHIP (Raw Vegan) by Julie

Serves 2 - 4

This is a very large, filling, smoothie designed to be eaten as a meal. One of the best digestive tonics around!

Ingredients:

> 1 young coconut (meat and juice)
>
> ¼ - ½ papaya (Roughly 2 cups of diced papaya chunks)
>
> 2 Tbsp. raw agave nectar (optional)
>
> mint garnish

Directions:

1. See *young coconut* in glossary for how to open one easily. Be sure to use all of the flesh and juice of the coconut, and place in blender.
2. Add papaya and agave to the blender. This is optional for those who like sweeter treats.
3. Whip everything together on the highest speed and blend until smooth.
4. Serve in beautiful tall glasses, and garnish with papaya seeds and mint sprigs (if you have them).

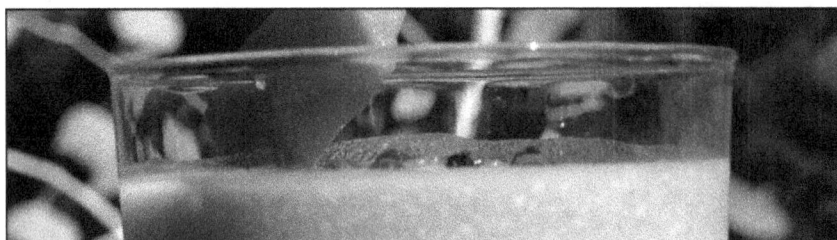

JUICY MORSEL: Papaya is loaded with digestive and anti-inflammatory enzymes! We like to rub the inner skin all over our own skin after the papaya is peeled. This helps get rid of dead skin cells, and also is a great way to use the skin before composting it. Just beware that if you lay down for a nap with papaya skin all over your face, you may be mistaken for a reptile if someone happens upon you and has no idea of your "practices"!

Papaya seeds taste like black pepper. Use these crunchy seeds for seasoning, or chew them up for a natural anti-parasitic intestinal cleanser!

COCONUT PROTEIN SHAKE (Raw Vegan) by Julie

Serves 2

Ingredients:

> 1 young coconut (meat and water)
>
> 1 red banana (or half organic yellow banana)
>
> 1 Tbsp. coconut oil or butter
>
> 2 Tbsp. raw protein powder (any nut powder will work)
>
> 1 tsp. probiotic powder (Julie uses All Flora from New Chapter)
>
> 2 heaping Tbsp. raw honey
>
> 3-6 ice cubes, depending on desired texture
>
> green powder, maca, or other superfood powder (optional)

Directions:

1. See *young coconut* in glossary for how to open one easily.
2. Blend all ingredients in regular blender or Vita-Mix for smoother shake.
3. Decorate with mint leaves or banana slice.

JUICY MORSEL: Young coconuts are almost always dipped in chemicals, numerous times, to preserve the white husk. You may find organic, chemical-free young coconuts at your local organic market. They will be small, light brown, and not as rough as the older dark brown coconuts. Organic coconuts are preferable, but not essential. Do the best you can!

LEAN GREEN SMOOTHIE (Raw Vegan) by Sarah

Serves 1-2

Ingredients:

3/4 cup RAW nut mylk or 1 young coconut (water and meat)

1 red banana (or half organic yellow banana)

1 Tbsp. dulse flakes

1 Tbsp. hemp seeds

2 leaves lacinto (dinosaur) kale

1 Tbsp. raw honey

3-6 ice cubes, depending on desired texture

Directions:

1. Blend all ingredients in traditional blender or Vita-Mix until smooth.
2. Serve in a glass with a sprinkle of extra hemp seeds on top as a nice garnish.

JUICY MORSEL: Hemp seeds are full of essential fatty acids. Don't let your mind run wild, and start conjuring up images of buttery flab hanging out of spandex leotards! Hemp seeds are an all-together different sort of fat source! They are not to be feared, as the fats contained in raw hemp are in the exact ratio of omega 3, 6, and 9 that is most optimal for the body. Enjoy the hemp, befriend it. Perhaps you could take it on a road trip!

NUT MYLK (Raw Vegan) by Sarah

Serves 4

Ingredients:

1 cup raw nuts of any kind (Sarah likes cashew best and Julie likes brazil nut or almond)

4 cups purified water

raw honey and cinnamon (optional)

Directions:

1. Soak nuts of choice in a bowl of purified water overnight, refrigerated. Use enough water to cover them.
2. Rinse nuts the following day in purified water.
3. Use ANY type of blender and blend nuts with 4 cups of water (4 to 1 ratio is best for all nut mylks). Blend until smooth.
4. Pour mixture into a sprout bag/nut mylk bag over a large bowl. Squeeze out all of the mylk until nut paste is the only thing left in the bag.
5. Pour mylk into glass jar. Keep refrigerated.
6. Optional: Add a few tablespoons of honey and some cinnamon for a sweet mylk. Sarah likes to put a cinnamon stick in there and leave overnight to flavor the mylk.
7. Shake mylk well before using, as it will separate while refrigerated. Stays fresh for about four days.
8. Reserve the leftover nut paste for use with Wanna B Chive Cheez recipe.

JUICY MORSEL: Store-bought nut mylks are full of toxic ingredients. They are pasteurized (cooked), which kills any benefit of the vitamins and fats.

Also, nut mylks from the store are full of toxic mineral rocks like calcium. Would you want to chew on a freshly mined piece of calcium carbonate? Neither would we! The FDA has done a fine job of scaring everyone into calcium paranoia; as if there is something wrong with the nut mylk that has no extra calcium poison. Hence, calcium is added to the mylk, to increase sales.

As if these two deterrents were not enough, most nut mylks have added sweeteners such as brown rice syrup. This syrup might sound like a healthful sweetener, but it is far from it. Think of how condensed and processed rice must get to produce a thick, syrupy sweetener; not too pretty! So don't fall for packaged mylks, make your own creamy delight! It is well worth the time and effort.

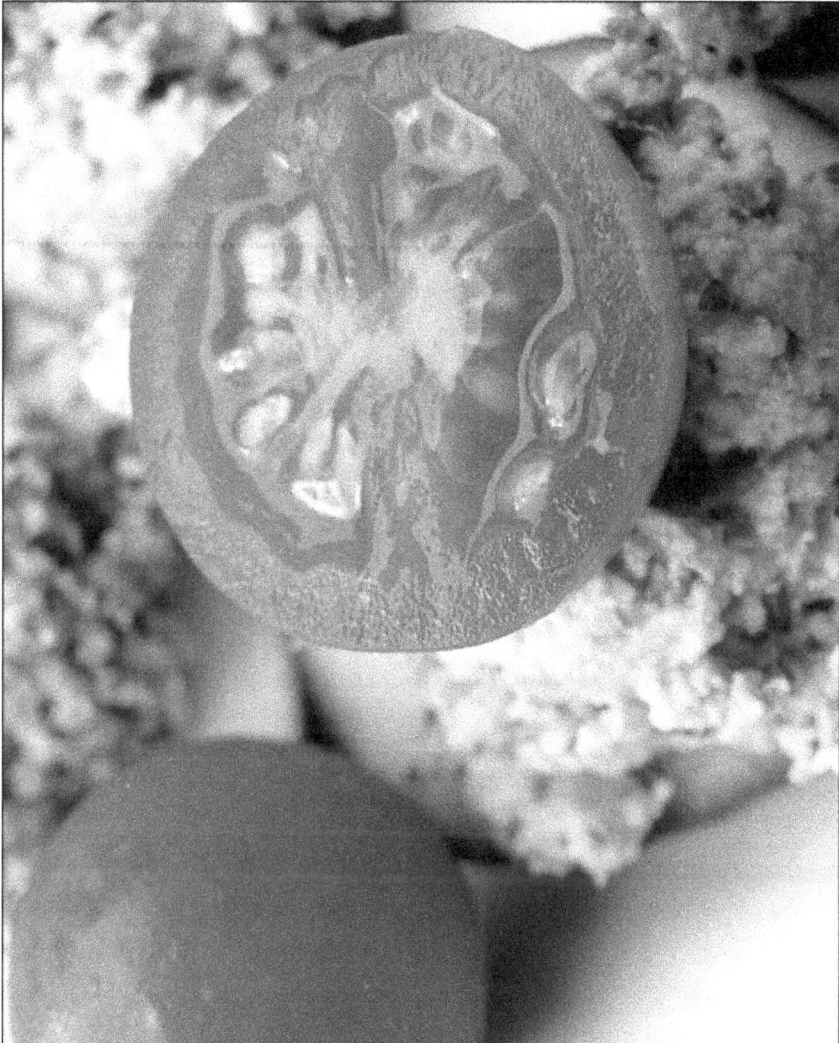

Dips
Appetizers
Photo: Wanna B Chive Cheez

SWEETLY STUFFED JALAPENOS (Cooked Vegetarian) by Sarah

Serves 4

Ingredients:

1 small yellow onion
1 gala apple (or any sweet baking apple)
8 jalapeno peppers
1 cup walnuts
3 oz. raw goat cheddar
3 Tbsp. organic unsalted butter
dash of sea salt

Directions:

1. Preheat oven to 375 degrees.
2. Finely dice the onion, walnuts, and apple. You may also do this in a food processor if you are short on time. Sarah is the queen of chopping and dicing, so she always does this by hand!
3. Add the butter to a sauté pan and melt.
4. Add the onion, apple, and walnut mixture and sauté until the onions and apples are sweet and soft. Add a dash of salt towards the end and taste. Mixture should be sweet with a slight saltiness to bring out flavors. Set mixture aside off heat when finished.
5. Slice the jalapenos lengthwise in half. Deseed them. (CAUTION: Seeds are very spicy and irritating to skin. We

recommend you do not touch your skin or eyes after deseeding.)

6. Grate the raw goat cheddar (more if you are a cheese-a-holic like some of us...hint hint).
7. Arrange the jalapeno halves in a baking dish/pan and fill them with the sautć mixture.
8. Cover and bake the stuffed jalapenos for approximately 30 minutes or until the peppers are soft.
9. Remove from oven and immediately top with a generous layer of the grated cheese. Let cool 5-10 minutes. This will mellow out the spice!

JUICY MORSEL: We know it is difficult to give up dairy. Raw goat cheese is great during those times when you swear you could suck the milk straight from the cow! Cow dairy is extremely hard to digest, even for those who feel no symptoms, and mucus forming. Delicious, eh?

Goat dairy is not nearly as rough on the body. Granted, you probably should not sit down with a brick-sized slab of goat cheese and call it a night. A nice slice or two a few times a week can be eaten without worry and can be part of a very healthful diet. Look for *raw* goat cheeses, as they will not be made from pasteurized goat milk and therefore much more healthful.

PERUVIAN OLIVE & RED PEPPER DIP (Raw Vegetarian) by Julie

Serves 4

Ingredients:

---

1 cup raw Peruvian oil-cured pitted olives

1 large or 2 small garlic cloves

2 Tbsp. chopped onion

½ red bell pepper

5 oz. raw feta cheese

2 Tbsp. olive oil

½ tsp. salt (optional)

Directions:

1. Coarsely chop the onion, garlic, olives, and pepper. Place in food processor.
2. Add the olive oil to food processor and blend well. This should be a smoother dip than olive tapenade, which tends to be chunkier.
3. Add the feta cheese and blend lightly until the cheese is mixed in.
4. Taste the dip and add salt if needed. The olives and feta tend to make the dip salty enough, but you will have to season to your liking.
5. Serve with veggies, raw crackers, or sprouted bread. Also makes a great spread for wraps! We like to spread this dip on some red Russian kale and then roll it up. Yummy in the tummy!

JUICY MORSEL: Olives have more mucus dissolving power than any other food. This is the best thing you can choose to eat if preparing a meal that contains dairy, as dairy tends to form mucus in the body.

Olives are also incredibly dense in minerals and beneficial fats. Consider these pitted pleasures an internal facial. Save some pennies at the spa and eat some olives instead.

BEANLESS MEDITERRANEAN HUMMUS (Raw Vegan) by Sarah

Serves 4

Ingredients:

1 medium zucchini
2 Tbsp. olive oil
1 tsp. sea salt
2 Tbsp. lemon juice
2 Tbsp. tahini
¼ tsp. cayenne
½ tsp. paprika
½ tsp. cumin

Directions:

1. Blend the zucchini first in a food processor until fairly smooth.
2. Add the rest of the ingredients to food processor and blend again until mixture is a smooth, thick dip texture. You may need to add more or less zucchini, depending on how thick you like your hummus to be.
3. This makes a wonderful spread for lettuce wraps, or a perfect dip to accompany a vegetable tray for parties!

JUICY MORSEL: Beans have enzyme inhibitors, which is why people often get gassy from them. If you sprout beans, they become more digestible, but never fully, and therefore are essentially an indigestible food. Beanless hummus is a much better option for ultimate health.

HOLY GUACAMOLE, I'M IN LOVE! (Raw Vegan) by Julie

Serves 4, or 2 guacamole addicts!*

Ingredients:

2 large Hass avocadoes

½ lemon, juiced well

1 cup loosely packed cilantro tops

1/8 red onion (about 3 Tbsp. when chopped)

1 small tomato

½ jalapeno pepper

½ tsp. garlic powder or 1 garlic clove

¾ tsp. sea salt

vegetables of choice for dipping

Directions:

1. Finely dice the onion, tomato, and jalapeno. If you are using a garlic clove, finely dice this as well. Set aside.
2. Loosely chop the cilantro tops. Set aside.
3. Mash the avocado "meat" in a medium bowl and leave fairly chunky.
4. Juice the lemon and add to avocado mash.
5. Add all of the chopped items, as well as the other listed items, to the avocado. Mash gently, but well, so that all of the flavors mix. Check to be sure the salt and garlic have been properly mixed, and add more to taste if you like.

6. Slice some vegetables of choice to use for dipping. We like zucchini and cucumber best because they make nice, crunchy chips! They are also relatively bland, which allows the guacamole flavor to come through.

*People generally swarm when I make this dish for parties. I think it's because I imagine how incredible the guacamole tastes when I make it...pure love!

JUICY MORSEL: There is an art to making guacamole. Most folks mash avocadoes with sour cream and salsa. This is cheating. Guacamole is all about chopping, dicing, and mashing things together slowly.

The avocado needs to stay thick and chunky; none of that soupy watered-down mess served so often at restaurants!

Why are folks so afraid of cilantro? Sometimes a sprig or two of this herb finds its way into the "guac." Come on! It's time to face the cilantro fear and really grab a fat handful. Chop, chop!

Then there is the garlic...oh sweet succulent garlic...diced so fine that it blends in and saturates each ingredient. Maybe I should write a book on guacamole. Have I lost you yet? It seems I am much more into the ravenous details of mashed avocadoes than the average Joe. Okay, I get it. I hear you loud and clear. Move on to the next recipe, Julie!

WANNA B CHIVE CHEEZ (Raw Vegan) by Julie

Serves 2

Ingredients:

¾ cup milked cashew paste (about 1 cup nuts before soaking and milking; see nut mylk instructions)

½ lemon

½ cup loosely packed chives

1 cup loosely packed Italian parsley

½ tsp. salt

1 zucchini or cucumber

cherry tomatoes (about a handful)

Directions:

1. Chop the parsley and chives coarsely. Add to food processor.
2. Juice the lemon and add to food processor.
3. Add the salt and cashew paste to the food processor and blend the mixture until smooth.
4. Slice the zucchini or cucumber into chip-like round discs. These can be topped with the cheez and half of a cherry tomato on top. *This cheez can also be used for wraps or veggie dip.*

JUICY MORSEL: Try this recipe with other herbs. Many of us have overgrown herbs in our garden, or herbs we never used up for the small recipes we bought them for. Throw the herbs into a nut paste and see what great combos you can come up with! How about tomato-oregano, cilantro-epazote, or parsley-lovage? At least you have some new herbs to look up and potentially plant. Gather up your pots and grow some culinary tasties.

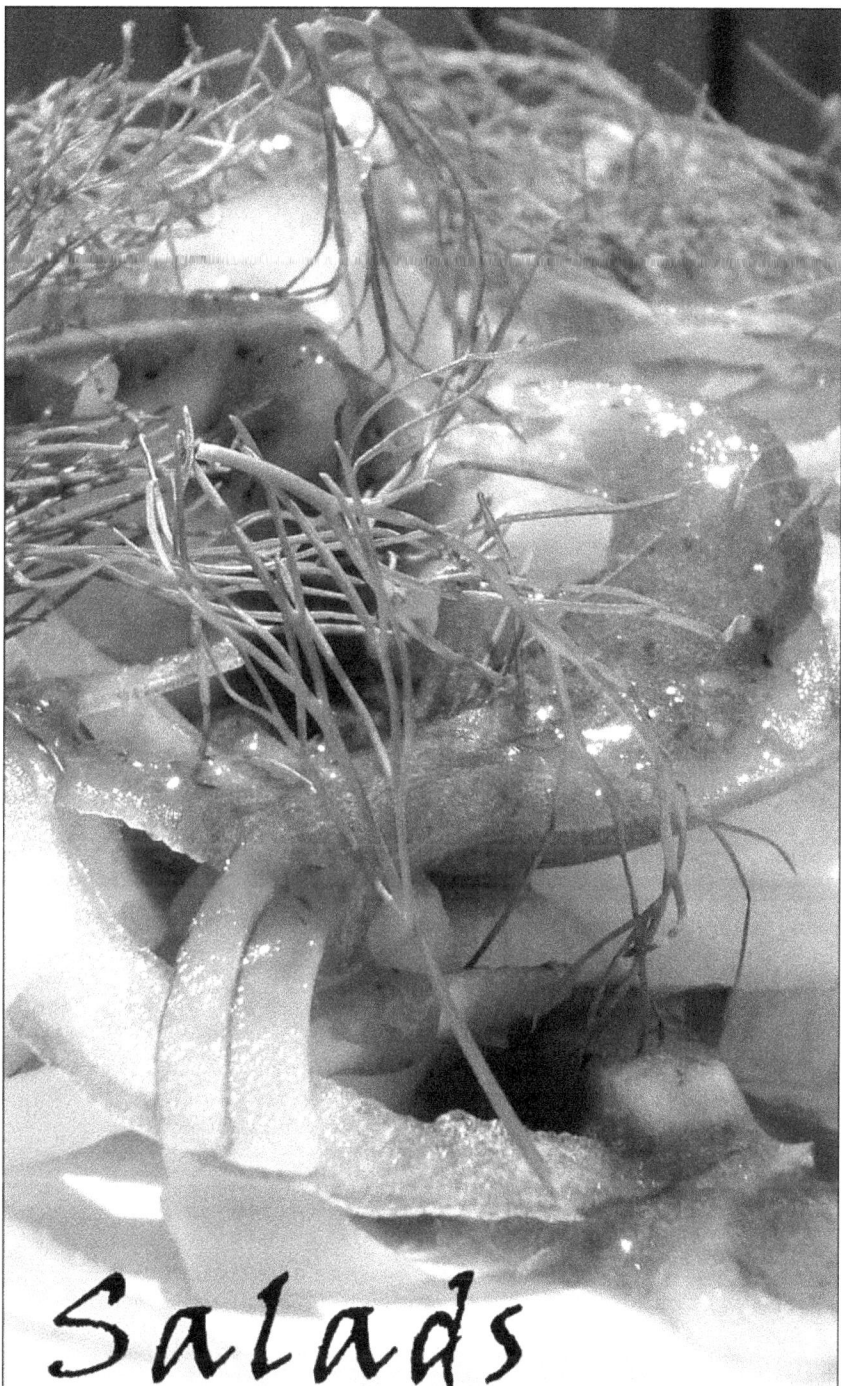

Salads

Photo: Fresh Fennel Salad

ASPARAGUS CUCUMBER SALAD (Raw Vegan) by Julie

Serves 2-4 (2 meals or 4 appetizer salads)

Ingredients:

15 thin asparagus stalks (or 10 thick ones)
2 small cucumbers
2 tsp. fresh chives
¼ red bell pepper
¼ cup parsley leaves

Directions:

1. Cut the top 2 inches off asparagus spears and set aside.
2. Slice the 2 cucumbers (skin on) into discs and arrange on a dinner-size plate or circular tray. Leave a small hole in the center.
3. Chop the asparagus BOTTOMS into ½ inch pieces and arrange neatly over the cucumbers.
4. Dice the chives and sprinkle over the cucumber and asparagus.
5. Place the asparagus tops in the center where the hole is. They should be standing on their bottoms and sort of leaning upon one another like little trees.
(See photo)
6. Take the parsley tops off of the stems and arrange them around the edge of the plate so that some of the green tops hang slightly off the side.
7. Slice the red pepper into thin long pieces and arrange them like sun rays coming from the asparagus. You may

want to tuck them under the asparagus tips slightly to hold them in place.

8. This salad is fresh and delicious as is. If you enjoy dressings, this salad is divine with the Herbed Ranch Dressing in our dressing section. It is the perfect, creamy, cool addition to the summer flavors in this salad. Drizzle the dressing over platter or use as a dip on the side.

JUICY MORSEL: Cucumbers are anti-inflammatory. Not only are they wonderful in salads, they make a great bland base for juices. Try juicing them with ginger and turmeric root for any inflammation issues.

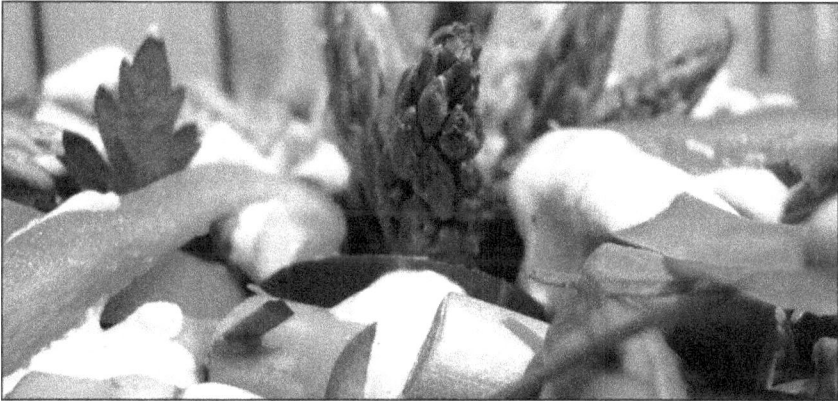

FRESH FENNEL SALAD (Raw Vegan) by Sarah

Serves 2

Ingredients:

½ small red onion

½ cup whole raspberries

1 medium fennel bulb with tops still attached

½ lemon

¼ cup pure water

¼ cup loosely packed parsley

1 Tbsp. raw honey

dash of sea salt

Directions:

1. Slice the fennel and onion into thin disc-like strips and set the green tops aside.
2. Chop the parsley and set aside.
3. Juice the lemon and add to blender.
4. Add the raspberries, salt, water, and honey to the blender and blend the mixture until smooth.
5. Place a layer of the sliced fennel on a plate with the onion evenly layered throughout.
6. Sprinkle the parsley over the top.
7. Drizzle the raspberry dressing over the salad. This salad is most beautiful on a white plate to show off the greens and red of the dressing. The dressing does not need to

smother everything; it should just be drizzled lightly over the salad and around the plate.

8. Top the salad with some delicate fennel tops. Just break off a few of the sprigs.

9. Serve as is. *If there is leftover dressing, save for dipping, other salads, or mixed fruit! If raspberries are out of season, this salad may be tossed with a bit of lemon juice, salt, and pepper.* Very refreshing and very light!

JUICY MORSEL: Got gas? Eat fennel. 'Nuff said!

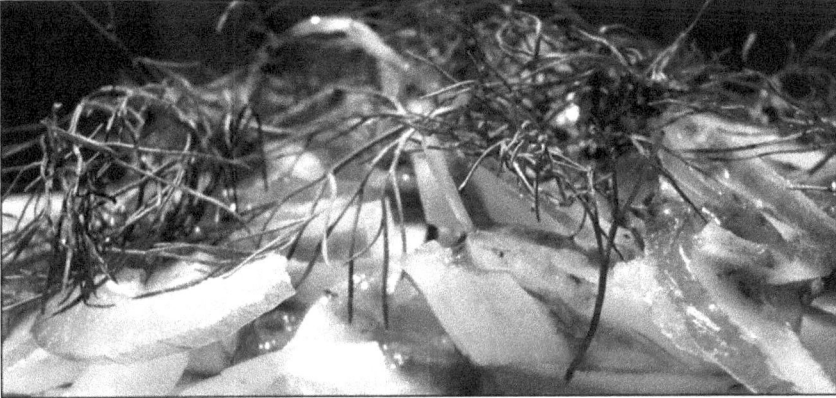

SARAH'S SPECIAL BLEND HERB SALAD (Raw Vegan)

Serves 2

Ingredients:

2 cups fresh basil (loose)

½ bunch Italian parsley tops

¼ medium red onion

1 handful cherry tomatoes

6 raw Botija olives or Kalamata olives

1 tsp. dulse flakes

2 Tbsp. olive oil

1 tsp. raw apple cider vinegar

1 lemon

pinch sea salt

pinch black pepper

Directions:

1. Reserve a large bowl for the salad.
2. Take basil leaves off stems and add to bowl.
3. Coarsely chop parsley tops and add.
4. Slice the onion thinly and add.
5. Pit and chop the olives. Add to bowl.
6. Sprinkle in the dulse.
7. Halve the tomatoes and lay them throughout the salad.

8. Combine the olive oil, lemon, vinegar, salt and pepper and pour over the salad.

9. Toss salad and dressing lightly in bowl and serve. *Raw goat cheddar slices compliment the salad nicely on the side. This is optional.*

JUICY MORSEL: Dulse is a seaweed rich in vitamins, minerals and iodine. I LOVE this sea vegetable plain in its leaf form! It is incredibly salty and is a great substitution for bacon cravings. Throw some dulse into a wrap or make a sprouted grain "DLT" with dulse, lettuce, and tomato.

Sometimes the salt in dulse is enough to get us through our bacon cravings. You need not gorge on dripping fatty tissue when you are lusty for bacon. If you prefer a crispy substitute, lightly toast the dulse in a frying pan with a drop of oil, and then add it to your meal. Eventually transition into the ability to eat it raw, as a snack, or sprinkled over meals as a condiment; that way the nutrition will not be cooked out.

SUPERFOOD SALAD (Raw Vegan) by Sarah

Serves 2-4 (2 salad meals or 4 appetizer salads)

Ingredients:

1 head romaine or red leaf lettuce
1 large tomato (we like Cherokee purple heirlooms best)
½ red onion
1 large carrot
1 cup baby arugula
¼ cup cacao nibs
½ cup goji berries
2 Tbsp. hemp seeds

Directions:

1. Rinse, dry, and chop the lettuce and arugula. Place in large salad bowl.
2. Grate the carrot and sprinkle over salad.
3. Thinly slice the tomato and onion. Arrange on top of salad.
4. Sprinkle the cacao nibs and gojis over the salad.
5. When served, sprinkle hemp seeds over the salad. Hemp seeds oxidize very quickly and are freshest straight out of the bag. This is why you should wait to add them to the salad until serving. This will preserve the volatile fats contained in them.

6. Choose any dressing from our dressing section, eat plain, or follow our favorite by tossing in a touch of raw apple cider vinegar and olive oil.

JUICY MORSEL: Cacao has become quite the controversial food. This raw form of chocolate has the highest antioxidant level of ANY known food! Cacao is unbelievably rich in magnesium and vitamin C. So what is the huff and puff all about?

There are active parts of cacao that burn out the adrenals over time because cacao is a stimulant. Liver toxification is another negative consequence of eating cacao. We hear this. We get it. We researched it. We know. Don't say we didn't warn you of the consequences of this horrible poison! Ha!

On a serious note, we think cacao can be great in small amounts. If you are getting off of coffee, cacao is a FANTASTIC substitution to get you through the transition. I must ask myself in this moment, "Which is healthier? A large caramel-mochacino-chocolicious-soy-latte-whipped-soycream-smoothie from the nearest coffee hut...or a few RAW cacao nibs thrown into my salad?" Point for me. Thank you. Now enjoy your superfood salad and then make my chocolate mousse recipe!

Sauces
Dressings

Photo: Herbed Ranch Dressing

AMOROUS AVOCADO WHIP (Raw Vegan) by Sarah

Makes 1 cup

Ingredients:

1 small head bok choy
1 large Hass avocado
¼ red bell pepper
½ jalapeno pepper
½ large lemon
½ cup pure water
½ tsp. cayenne
½ tsp. cumin powder
pinch sea salt

Directions:

1. Wash the bok choy, chop into salad size pieces, and set aside to drain.
2. A blender works best, but you may also make the dressing in a food processor. Peel and deseed the avocado and add to blender.
3. Add the water to blender.
4. Remove seeds from peppers, cut into pieces, and add to blender.
5. Juice the lemon and add to blender.
6. Add the seasonings and salt to taste and blend well until creamy.

7. Mix the avocado whip by hand with the bok choy. Serve at room temperature or let the bok choy and avocado whip chill separately in the refrigerator, and serve chilled. Other lettuces may be substituted, but the mild and crisp nature of bok choy works best with the flavors.

JUICY MORSEL: Bok choy is full of calcium. Ditch the rock pills and start chewing some of this crunchy treat!

CHEEZ for MAC N CHEEZ (Raw Vegan) by Julie

Serves 2

This cheez sauce is most like Velveeta or nacho cheese consistency. Use as a dip or filling for wraps, too! May also be used with cooked corn chips for those transitioning off dairy and not yet completely raw. Also a great veggie dip for kids!

Ingredients:

¼ cup pine nuts

¼ cup truly raw cashews

¼ red bell pepper

lemon wedge

¼ cup olive oil

¾ tsp. sea salt

2 Tbsp. Brewer's Yeast

few sprigs fresh parsley

Directions:

1. Blend cashews and pine nuts first in any type of food processor.
2. Add rest of ingredients EXCEPT PARSLEY to the nut paste and blend thoroughly.
3. Mix sauce into zucchini noodles or kelp noodles.

Kelp noodles may be chopped up to look like macaroni size. Found in most health food stores, they are best when lightly salted with a squeeze of lemon. Allow to sit 20 minutes or more.

Zucchini noodles can be made by using a carrot peeler to make long, thin slices of zucchini. Lightly salt them and allow them to sweat for a few minutes before adding cheez sauce.

4. Garnish with a few sprigs of parsley.

JUICY MORSEL: When you purchase Brewer's Yeast, it is best to find one that does not say "Nutritional Yeast." True Brewer's Yeast is in its original form without added B vitamins. The vitamins added are isolates, in toxic forms to the body. These isolates bear no resemblance to natural B vitamins from fruits and vegetables. Nature is smart. There are loads of B vitamins in Brewer's Yeast. You do not need added vitamins, especially the isolated forms that have no relation to food. Check the ingredients list; if the only thing listed is Brewer's Yeast, go with it!

DELECTABLE DILL DRESSING (Raw Vegan) by Julie

Makes about 1 ½ cups

Ingredients:

½ cup olive oil

½ cup raw apple cider vinegar

3 Tbsp. Bragg's Liquid Aminos

2 Tbsp. Nama Shoyu

2 Tbsp. tahini

2 Tbsp. red miso

3 Tbsp. dry dill or ¼ cup fresh chopped dill

1-2 garlic cloves, minced

dash black pepper

Directions:

1. Use a garlic crusher to mince the garlic.
2. Chop the dill if using fresh dill.
3. Add all ingredients to a glass jar.
4. Shake well and let the flavors blend in the refrigerator for a few hours. This dressing will hold up well for at least a week. If the ingredients thicken and separate, shake vigorously or add a tablespoon or two of water.
5. Toss into a salad of your choice or use as a dipping sauce for vegetables.

JUICY MORSEL: The word dill comes from Norse "dilla." This word meant "to lull." Adding dill to a variety of things helps keep us calm. You can also brew any leftover fresh dill from this recipe into a wonderful tea.

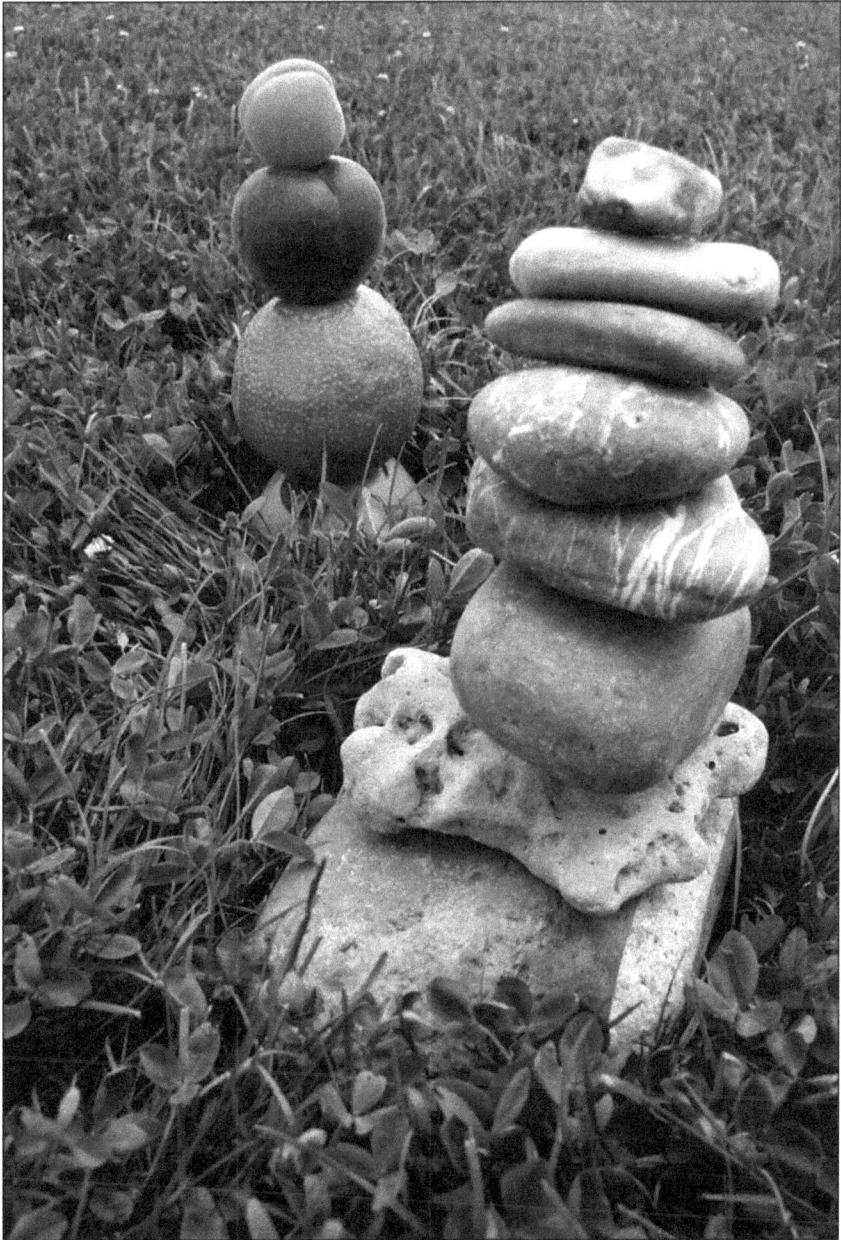

HERBED RANCH DRESSING (Raw Vegan) by Julie

Makes 1 cup

Ingredients:

2/3 cup pure water

½ lemon

2/3 cup cashews

1 Tbsp. pine nuts

¼ cup fresh parsley tops

1/8 red bell pepper

1 tsp. fresh chives

10 small basil leaves

2 small garlic cloves

¾ tsp. sea salt

Directions:

1. Blend the water, pine nuts, and cashews in blender until fairly smooth.
2. Coarsely chop the red pepper, chives, garlic, and parsley tops. Add them to the blender.
3. Blend again until fairly smooth.
4. Juice the lemon and add to blender.
5. Add the basil and salt.
6. Blend on high until mixture is smooth and creamy. Taste and adjust salt or herbs to your preference.

This is a very versatile dressing! We created it to be paired with our Asparagus Cucumber Salad, but it may also be used in wraps or as a mild dairy-free dipping sauce for veggies. Kids love this one because it is mild, fresh, and has the consistency of real veggie dip!

JUICY MORSEL: Everyone loves dips and dressings. These food additions have become a necessity. The only time I can remember seeing someone not put dressing on their salad, was when a friend of mine became anorexic, and did not want the extra calories.

It's amazing to think about the fact that no one really eats plain salad...EVER! I am taking this moment to encourage you to enjoy two extremes. Drench your salad in the saucy ranchiness above; then the next day attempt to eat a plain salad. What do the red peppers, baby lettuces, and onion really taste like? Ask yourself if you really must drench everything, or if you can adjust to appreciating the gifts our taste buds get from each plain vegetable. You just may surprise yourself, and start eating onions as if they are apples!

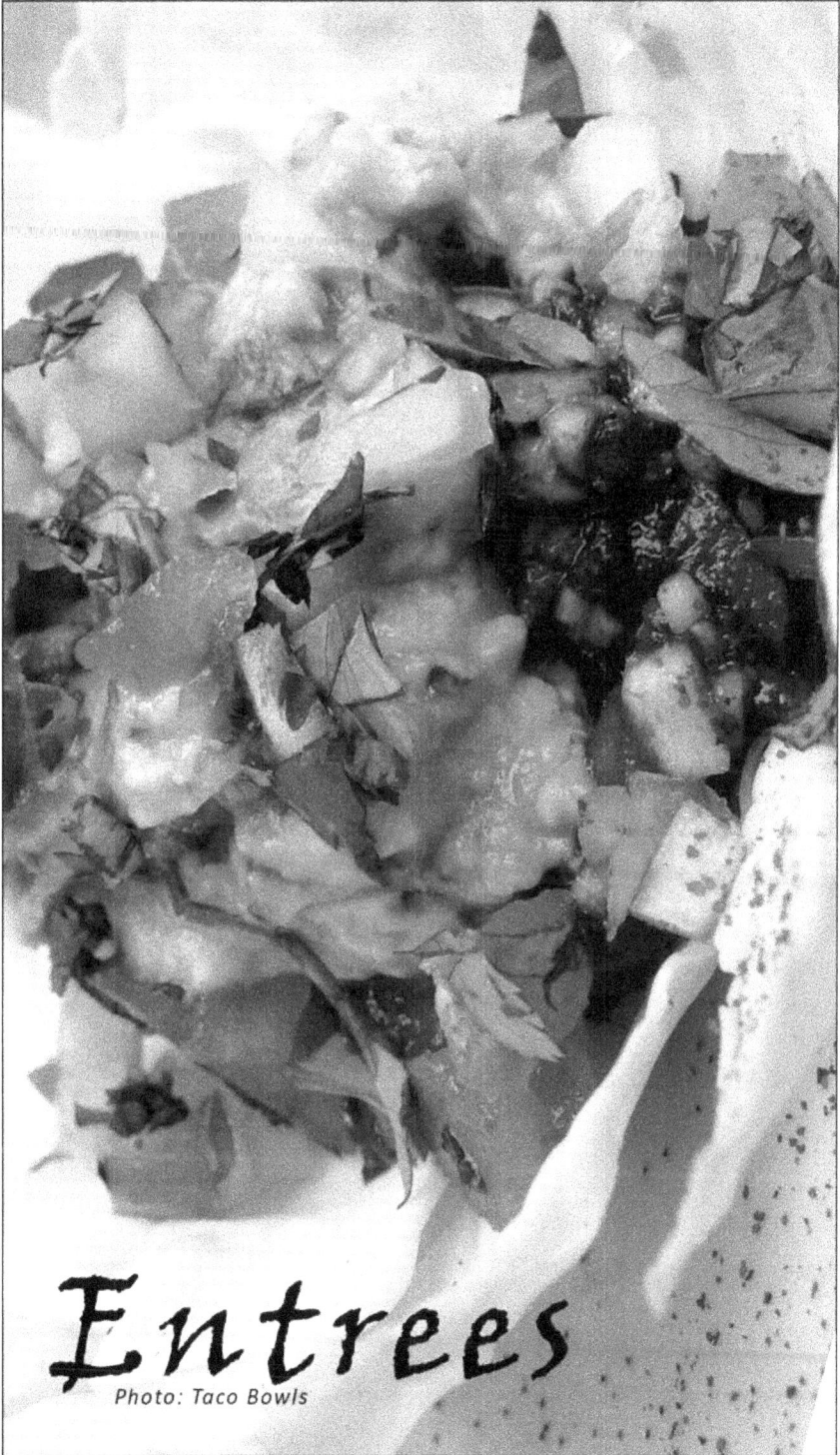

Entrees

Photo: Taco Bowls

NO-NOODLES-NECESSARY LASAGNE (Cooked Vegetarian)

by Sarah *Serves 6-8*

Ingredients:

1 medium eggplant

3 small to medium zucchinis

8 roma tomatoes

2 cups spinach

1 yellow onion

6 oz. white mushrooms

6 garlic cloves

1 cup loose fresh oregano

1 ½ cups loose fresh basil

½ bunch Italian parsley

12 oz. whole milk ricotta cheese

4 oz. shredded parmesan cheese

12 oz. whole mozzarella

3 Tbsp. olive oil

¼ cup water

sea salt

pinch black pepper

Directions:

Eggplant and Zucchini prep:

1. Preheat oven to 350 degrees.
2. Slice the eggplant into round ¼ inch slices and slice zucchinis lengthwise into 1/8 inch slices. Lay both onto baking sheets and dust with sea salt. Allow to sweat while working on the sauce below.

Sauce prep: (Sarah does not pre-chop everything and then add to pan all at once. She enjoys the process of each item being added to the pan slowly, as each one is chopped. The thicker items are added first, like onions and garlic. Then she adds the more delicate items, such as spices and herbs. This sequence allows the flavors to naturally blend and fold into one another. As you complete each step below, add the ingredient to the saucepan after it is chopped.)

1. Use large saucepan and place over medium heat. Add 2 Tbsp. olive oil to pan.
2. Chop yellow onion and the garlic cloves and add to pan. Allow to begin glazing.
3. Coarsely chop mushrooms and add.
4. Finely chop parsley and add. Stir the mixture as each item is added.
5. Finely chop basil and add.
6. Finely chop oregano and add. Turn heat to low and stir briefly.
7. Blend 4 roma tomatoes in food processor and add to sauce.
8. Dice 4 more roma tomatoes and add.

9. Turn heat back up to medium and mix in diced tomatoes. Let simmer.

AT THIS POINT: Pat dry the zucchini and eggplant with cloth or towel. Flip over and lightly salt again. Allow to sweat.

10. Lightly chop spinach and add.
11. Add ¼ cup water and stir.
12. Cover and let simmer 5 minutes.
13. Add 1 ½ tsp. salt, pinch black pepper, and stir. Turn off heat.

Baking:

1. Take out 11x7x1.5 inch (or larger) Pyrex dish and set on top of baking sheet to collect any juices. Grease the Pyrex with 1 Tbsp. olive oil.
2. Pat dry zucchini and eggplant.
3. Cover bottom of Pyrex with 1 layer eggplant so no holes show.
4. Add thin layer of sauce.
5. Add layer of ricotta, using entire container.
6. Thinly slice ½ of the mozzarella and cover the ricotta.
7. Add a layer of zucchini so that cheese it covered.
8. Add layer of sauce and smooth over the zucchini.
9. Lay the remaining eggplant over zucchini. If there is any leftover zucchini or eggplant, it may be sautéed with any leftover juices or sauce as a side dish.
10. Add thin layer of sauce over zucchini.
11. Top with rest of mozzarella, thinly sliced.
12. Bake 45 minutes at 350 degrees, or until cheese is lightly browned.

13. Top with shredded parmesan and let stand 10 minutes before serving. NOTE: This is a little crispier than regular noodle lasagna, which tends to turn into mush. Our zucchini and eggplant stays slightly crisp, and therefore provides a slightly different texture to the average noodle lasagna. This is a perfectly delicious difference. Vegetables were made to be crunchy, not wimpy!

JUICY MORSEL: We could have made lasagna with good-old-fashioned wheat noodles. Sarah is sensitive to wheat. (Okay, maybe a bit more than sensitive; she gets puffy and likes to take sixteen hour hibernation naps!) Wheat is also not the best ingredient for keeping the bloodstream clean. The gluten in wheat tends to clog up the bloodstream, as if it was a form of glue.

Perhaps lasagna is one of your all-time favorite meals. Now you can enjoy a vegetarian version, eliminating the meat and the wheat. Zucchini is as mild-tasting as noodles, soaks up the flavors, and eliminates the wheat allergy factor. Try using zucchini as a substitute for any bland ingredient from a mainstream recipe. You will add vitamins and minerals, while lowering allergy and toxification problems!

LIMEY LEEK WRAPS (Cooked Vegan) by Sarah

Serves 4

Ingredients:

1 Romaine or red leaf lettuce head

1 small head cauliflower

1 medium parsnip

1 large leek

1 medium tomato

2 limes

2-3 inches ginger (skin on)

6 garlic cloves

1 large jalapeno pepper

½ cup cilantro

2 Tbsp. olive oil

1 tsp. salt

½ tsp. cayenne powder

pinch black pepper

Directions:

1. Steam the cauliflower and parsnip until soft and mashable. This may be done while you are preparing the rest below.

2. Place a wok over very low heat and add the olive oil. The pan should warm as you prepare the items below.
3. Grate the ginger on the grater side that has medium holes. Add ginger to wok.
4. Thinly slice the garlic and add to wok.
5. Remove the seeds from the jalapeno, dice it, and add to wok.
6. Chop the leek into small pieces (cross-sections). If they are not small pieces, lightly dice them again after the whole leek is cut. Add the leeks to a strainer and rinse extremely well! They generally are covered in dirt and sand. Then add them to the wok.
7. Turn heat to medium and stir frequently until leeks are soft, sweet, and tender. Set aside when done.
8. Check on the steamed items. When soft, mash them in large bowl like you would mash potatoes.
9. Add the leek sauté to the bowl and mix well.
10. Add the salt, cayenne, black pepper and stir.
11. Juice the lime and add to bowl. Stir well and taste. Add more spices or salt if needed.
12. Dice the tomato and cilantro. Set aside.
13. Remove lettuce leaf, rinse if needed, and lay flat on plate.
14. Spread about a handful of the leek mixture into the middle of the lettuce leaf, and top with diced tomatoes and cilantro.
15. Squeeze a small amount of fresh lime juice over the toppings, and cover with another lettuce leaf. This may be eaten as is, like a sandwich (although a bit messy), or you may wrap the bottom half in a paper towel or deli paper, to keep everything intact.

To compliment the lime and cool down the spiciness, add a touch of Wanna B Chive Cheez. (See recipe)

JUICY MORSEL: Leeks are a hidden treasure not appreciated by most. When we ask someone what they are having for din-din, how often do they respond, "A nice leek sauté"?

Rarely, if ever. I have no recollection of my family ever cooking with leeks. Sarah's mom has introduced them to me, and I can't get enough! Leeks are like onions, but sweeter and milder. This vegetable can also be used in its raw form. Try leeks in dips or chop them up in a salad.

Why bother with leeks? These tasty cousins of the onion are loaded with potassium and manganese, and are cardio-protective. What's not to love?

STUFFED MUSHROOMS (Cooked Vegan) by Sarah

Serves 3

Ingredients:

4 small purple potatoes

1 medium red potato

6 small-medium portabella mushrooms

½ red onion

2 stalks celery

2 handfuls baby carrots

½ bunch Italian parsley

¾ inch ginger (with skin)

3 large garlic cloves

2 cups rice cooking wine or chardonnay

2 tsp. sea salt

3 Tbsp. olive oil

1/8 tsp. cayenne powder

pinch black pepper

1 jalapeno pepper for spice (optional)

Directions:

Potato Prep:

1. Cut all potatoes into pieces, and boil them until soft and mashable.
2. Strain the potatoes when soft.
3. Mash with 1 tsp. sea salt, pinch black pepper, 1 Tbsp. olive oil, and 1/8 tsp. cayenne.

Vegetable Prep:

1. Take stems out of portabellas and add to food processor.
2. Place the mushroom caps upside down in a baking dish. (Pyrex is best)
3. Add following to food processor: onion, ginger, garlic, chopped celery, carrots, parsley, and optional jalapeno for spice.
4. Process the above with mushroom stems in food processor until chopped, but not pureed.

Sauté Prep:

1. Add 2 Tbsp. olive oil to wok on medium heat and let it warm.
2. Put veggie mixture into wok and sauté until onions soften, stirring occasionally.
3. Add 1 tsp. sea salt when nearly done with sauté.
4. Add mashed potatoes to wok and mix everything with heat off.
5. Preheat the oven to 375 degrees.

Assembly and Baking:

1. Stuff the mushrooms abundantly (1-2 inches over rim) with the veggie/potato mixture. Round them off like small mountains and leave them in baking dish.
2. Drip 2 cups rice cooking wine over mushrooms VERY slowly so the sauté absorbs the wine.
3. Cover with tinfoil or lid.
4. Let mushrooms bake until soft about 25 minutes. At this point they should be re-basted, and the lid or foil should be removed.
5. Heat oven to 475 degrees and bake as is for 15 minutes to allow tops to crisp up.

6. Let stand 10-15 minutes and serve warm. The mixture will look watery, but as the potatoes cool, they will begin to soak up the extra juices. This thick gravy may be poured over the stuffed mushrooms. Mmm!

JUICY MORSEL: Celery is full of organic salt! If you add bits of celery to your meals, you will need less salt for seasoning. Organic sodium is more healthful for the body. My Grandma uses celery leaves in her marinara sauce and it adds an indescribable flavor! Celery leaves are perfectly edible. We are trained to eat the stalks and throw away the leaves, but they should be kept for seasoning and juicing.

Celery juice is an excellent choice for heavy exercise days due to the great salt and mineral base it contains. Your mission, should you choose to accept it (please note the intense, edge-of-your-seat background music), is to do a round of push-ups and then enjoy some fresh celery juice. Three sets, baby! GO, GO, GO!

CREAMY MARINARA (Raw Vegan) by Julie

Serves 2

Ingredients:

1 cup truly raw cashews
1 medium heirloom tomato
½ diced roma tomato
2 zucchini
3-4 sundried tomatoes soaked in olive oil (Julie likes even more tomatoes...add to your own liking)
1 cup loosely packed basil
2 small garlic cloves
squeeze of lemon
½ tsp. salt (or more, depending on your taste buds)
extra fresh basil for garnish

Directions:

Zucchini Noodles: (Use 2 shallow, wide serving bowls with rims or 2 medium plates.)

1. Use carrot/potato peeler to shave zucchini into "pasta" noodles. One zucchini per dish.
2. Fluff them and dust with salt very lightly to let them soften. These will be the base. You may have some zucchini cores left, which may be set aside for salads or dipping vegetables.

Marinara Sauce:

1. In food processor, blend cashews until somewhat chunky.
2. Add basil, garlic, lemon, heirloom tomato, sundried tomatoes, and salt; blend until creamy.
3. Check zucchini noodles and if there is any water at the bottom of bowls, pour out and wipe bowls neatly.
4. Lay the creamy marinara over the noodles in a straight line down the middle.
5. Dice the roma tomato and sprinkle over the sauce.
6. Chop a few basil leaves and crumble over roma tomatoes and around the edge of zucchini pasta. Serve as is. This meal is most beautiful on a plain, white plate to show off the incredible reds and greens.

JUICY MORSEL: While garnish seems like an unnecessary addition to meals, it is great for so many reasons! First, garnish adds beauty to bland, colorless dishes.

We also think that garnish is like a sneak peek into the meal you are about to eat. The basil and tomato in the above recipe give hints about the flavors to come, so we can allow our mouths to water (which begins digestion).

Lastly, garnish is a wonderful, easy way to get some extra dense minerals added to your meal. Herbs and spices most often used as garnish are loaded with nutrition. These herbs also taste better mixed into a meal, versus by themselves, for those people transitioning into some of the intense vegetable tastes. Garnish up!

PESTO PASTA (Raw Vegan) by Sarah

Serves 2

Ingredients:

1 cup kelp noodles (found in refrigerated section of health food stores)

¼ cup truly raw cashews

½ cup fresh basil

¼ cup fresh Italian parsley

1 garlic clove

4 Tbsp. olive oil

lemon wedge(s)

½ tsp. sea salt

Directions:

1. Rinse kelp noodles with purified water and gently towel dry to collect extra water.
2. Squeeze the lemon wedge(s) over the noodles and dust with a sprinkle of salt. Set aside in a bowl to marinate while you make the pesto sauce.
3. Place the cashews in a food processor and blend well until fairly smooth.
4. Add the basil, parsley, salt, garlic, and olive oil to the food processor, and blend well with the cashews.

5. Toss the pesto with the noodles you set aside. This dish may be served immediately, or left in the refrigerator for a couple of hours, to soften the noodles and blend the flavors optimally. Garnish with fresh lemon wedges.

JUICY MORSEL: Basil is available in bountiful forms. One of our favorites is holy basil. While this favorite is not often found in the U.S., fresh, the tea is quite common now. This form of basil is a dual-directional herb, which means it balances the body based on what your body needs in the moment.

For example, if you are very stressed out and full of anxious energy, holy basil will mellow you out by lowering cortisol levels (your stress hormone). If you wake up exhausted, holy basil can perk you up and increase alertness!

This duality is where the magic of nature reveals itself. Holy basil has the power to read our bodies, know what they need, and create an effect based on that need. Simply exquisite.

PORTABELLA PIZZAS (Raw Vegan/Vegetarian) by Julie
Serves 4

Ingredients (Pizza base and toppings):

4 large portabella mushrooms

¼ small onion

½ tomato

12 Kalamata olives

fresh basil leaves (a few sprigs)

raw goat cheese (optional)

Marinade Ingredients:

¼ cup olive oil

½ lemon, squeezed

½ cup water

½ tsp. sea salt

1 tsp. dry parsley

1 tsp. dry oregano

dash black pepper

Pizza Sauce Ingredients:

½ cup sun dried tomatoes

1 medium to large garden tomato

1 large garlic clove

1 ½ Tbsp. olive oil

1 Tbsp. dry basil

2 Tbsp. dry oregano

1 Tbsp. dry parsley

½ tsp. sea salt, or more, to taste

Directions:

Mushroom Directions:

1. Cut the stems off the portabellas and set them in the refrigerator for later.
2. Mix all marinade ingredients, by hand, in a bowl.
3. Pour the marinade over the 4 portabella tops. This works best if you use a non-metal dish, such as a glass Pyrex baking dish. The portabellas should be upside down, so that they hold some of the marinade.
4. Place the portabellas in the refrigerator (covered) and allow them to marinate for 4-8 hours. This marinade is very light and designed to just add some moisture, not to fully flavor the mushrooms. Check them after an hour or two and baste with the marinade again.

Sauce Directions:

1. Place sundried tomatoes and the garden tomato in a food processor and blend until somewhat chunky.
2. Add the rest of the sauce ingredients to the food processor and blend well.
3. Place the pizza sauce in the refrigerator, to let the flavors blend, while the portabellas marinate. *If you prefer a room temperature sauce, make this sauce about 30 minutes before the portabellas are done marinating. Allow the sauce to sit at room temperature as you do the toppings.*

Assembly Directions:

1. Slice the portabella stems into thin round circles.
2. Slice the onions into very thin slivers.
3. Slice ½ tomato into delicate slices.
4. Dice the Kalamata olives and remove any pits.
5. Remove basil leaves from the stems.
6. Place the portabellas on a serving tray so that the smooth top is face down.
7. Take the pizza sauce and spread a generous amount within each portabella mushroom base.
8. Layer the sliced ingredients over the sauce in the following order to build your pizza toppings: tomatoes, mushrooms, goat cheese (optional), onions, basil, and olives. Garnish the tray with basil leaves. (optional)

JUICY MORSEL: Portabella mushrooms are often contaminated with mold from sitting in boxes for weeks. Check the mushrooms before purchasing, and if there is any white or dark fungus-looking growth on the mushrooms, move on to the next store.

If the mushrooms have a little dirt on them, do not worry; this is fine. Mushrooms grow in dirt, and we should expect that they might not be perfectly clean. However, do not hesitate to be proactive with the produce department(s) where you shop. Ask the manager to buy smaller quantities that sell quicker, and therefore lessen the chance of mold.

You can also ask for your own case of portabellas and share them with another family or two. This allows the mushrooms to go straight from the produce shipper to you, without sitting on a shelf. Sometimes stores will offer case discounts, too!

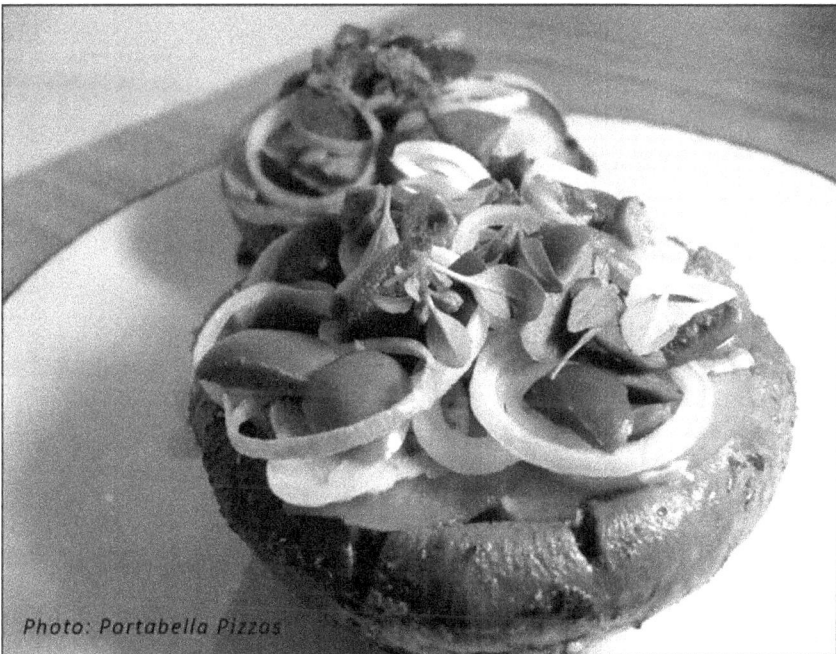

Photo: Portabella Pizzas

TACO BOWLS (Raw Vegan) by Julie

Serves 3 (2 tacos each)

Ingredients:

1 large portabella mushroom
1 medium tomato
1 head purple or white cabbage
½ large zucchini or 1 small one
¼ red onion
½ cup cilantro
2 small garlic cloves
¼ cup olive oil
2 tsp. unsalted taco seasoning
¾ tsp. sea salt (or to taste)
1/8 tsp. cayenne powder

Directions:

Taco "Meat":

1. Finely chop the mushroom, zucchini, and garlic.
2. Mix in salt, taco seasoning, cayenne, and olive oil.
3. Set aside to let flavors blend.

Toppings:

1. Chop the following by hand and leave in separate piles: onion, cilantro, and tomato.

Assembly:

1. Carefully peel off 6 leaves of cabbage. These will be the "bowls" for the tacos. Sometimes the leaves rip, and you can nestle 2 leaves inside of each other to create a stronger bowl. *The trick to getting the leaves off without ripping is to cut the leaves at the base of the cabbage head. They should then pull right off.*
2. Fill each of the 6 bowls with a generous scoop of taco "meat."
3. Top each taco with a layer of onions, followed by tomatoes and cilantro. You may need larger amounts if you like loads of toppings in your tacos. Adjust as you like.
4. Place 2 tacos on each plate and savor the juiciness! Don't be afraid to get messy...there will be lots of drips and dribbles of raw flavor! *Top with Julie's Holy Guacamole, I'm in Love!* (optional)

JUICY MORSEL: A large part of transitioning into raw food, is the appearance of the things we eat. The raw taco bowls are a perfect example of a recipe that looks, smells, and feels like a taco that would have meat in it. The olive oil, taco seasoning, and mushrooms create gravy that seeps out of the bowls and onto the plate. When I first sampled this recipe to a friend (who is not vegetarian), she claimed, "Wow! That really looks like the oily gravy that drips out of tacos!"

Not all of us need taco filling that looks like meat. Eventually, the thought of meat begins to turn the stomach. But for people just coming off of cooked food and moving into a vegetarian diet, these recipes can be a lifesaver! The visual appeal is the first thing to grab our attention.

We recommend this meal for people who are battling meat cravings, as well as people who can't eat a pile of greens yet without dreaming of patchouli-saturated hippies meditating in caves. So-called "rabbit food" is an acquired taste after years of cooked and seasoned foods. This is perfectly understandable! Enjoy some of our more savory recipes that mimic mainstream eating, until you can focus more on the pure tastes of plain fruits and vegetables.

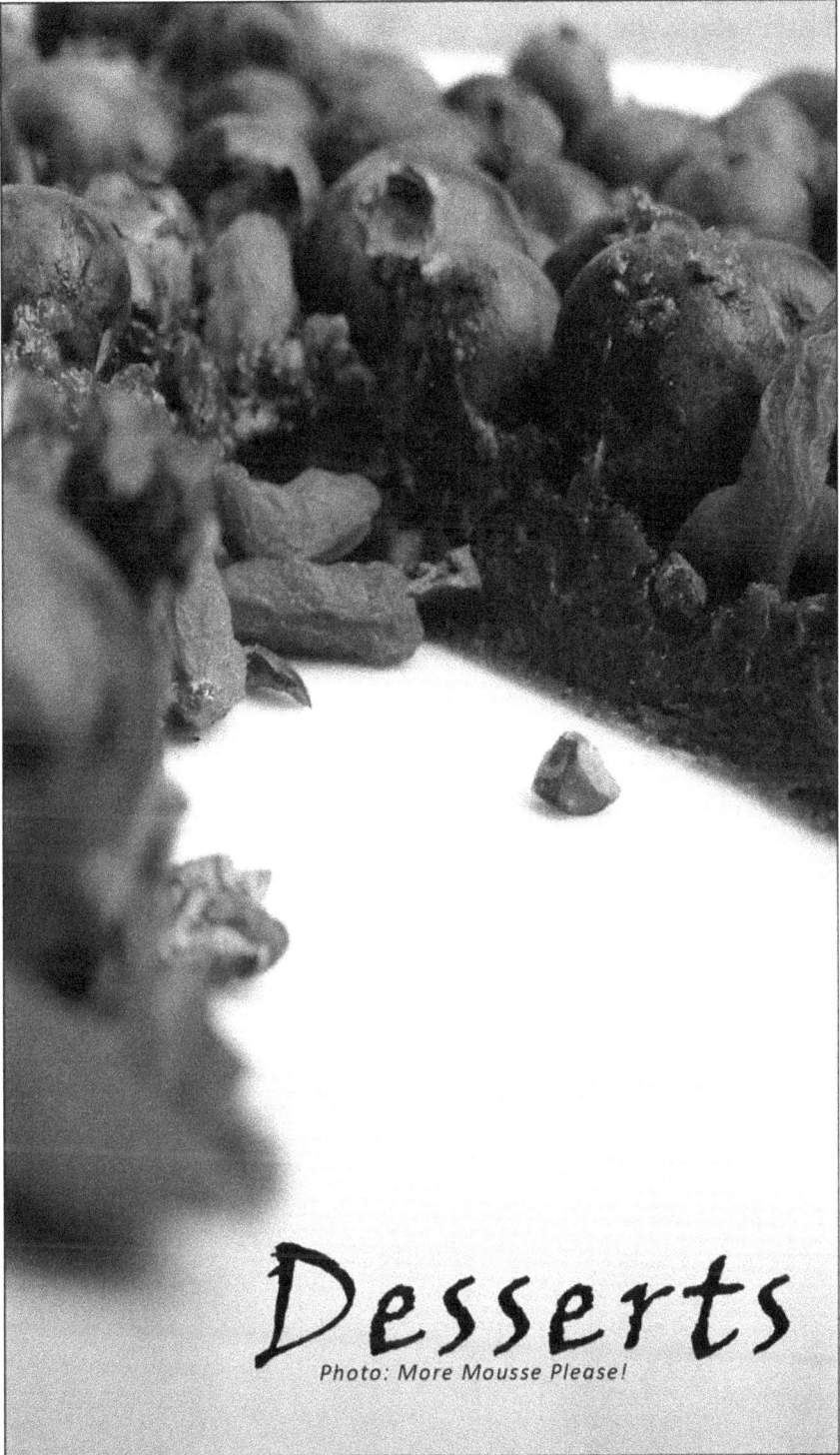

Desserts
Photo: More Mousse Please!

INCAN DREAM COOKIES (Raw Vegan) by Julie

Serves 4

Ingredients:

1 cup truly raw cashews
½ cup pine nuts
½ cup lucuma powder
1 Tbsp. raw honey
1 Tbsp. purified water
dash sea salt
Garnish: a few goji berries or cacao beans

Directions:

1. Blend the cashews in food processor until relatively fine.
2. Add the rest of the ingredients, except garnish, to the food processor and blend well.
3. Check texture of the cookie dough by pinching some to see if it sticks together fairly well. If it falls apart easily, add a touch more water.
4. Form the dough into 1 inch balls (or small mountains). Makes 8-10 cookies.
5. Garnish the cookies with a cacao bean or goji berry pressed into the top of the cookie.

JUICY MORSEL: Lucuma powder is the closet flavor we have found to caramel. You can add this treat to smoothies, juices, or desserts to create a very rich flavor.

Our dream is to have our own lucuma tree one day, so we can enjoy the fruit as it exists in nature. Until then, the powder is a great source not only of flavor, but also of iron, calcium, and beta-carotene.

The lucuma fruit was termed "Gold of the Incas" in South America. Now we know why! The flavor alone is worth its weight in gold. Perhaps you have been to South America and enjoyed some lucuma ice-cream, which is the equivalent of our chocolate ice-cream...very common and readily available! Speaking of which, I think I will go make a new raw food recipe for lucuma ice-cream. Delish!

LEMON TART (Raw Vegan) by Julie

Serves 4

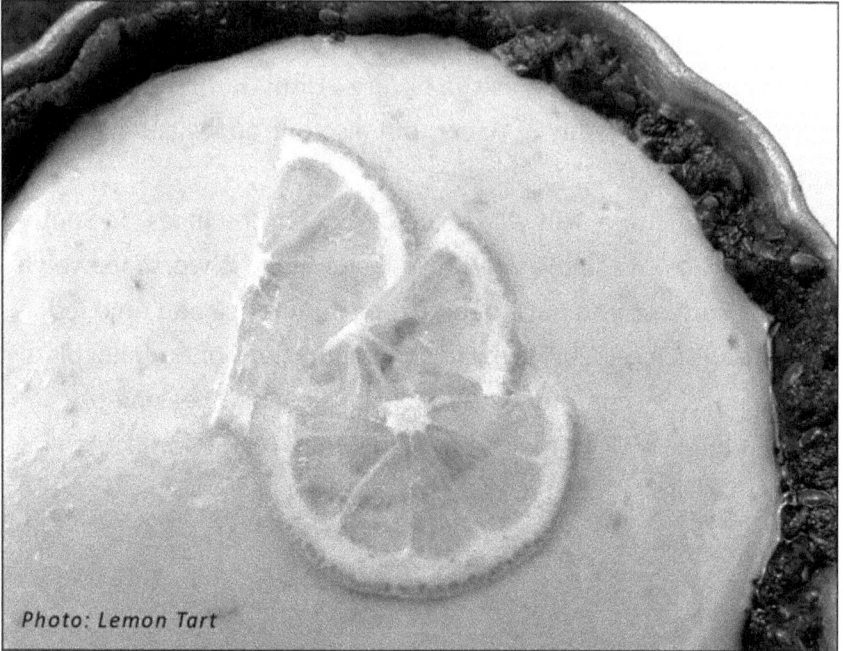

Photo: Lemon Tart

Crust Ingredients:

1 cup raw walnuts
1 Tbsp. coconut butter
½ tsp. cinnamon
2 Tbsp. raw agave nectar
1 Tbsp. flax seed (sprouted is best)
pinch sea salt

Topping ingredients:

1/3 cup pine nuts

2 Tbsp. raw honey (less or more, depending on tartness desired)

1 Tbsp. coconut butter (oil will work as well)

1 lemon, juiced

Directions:

Crust:

1. Blend walnuts in food processor until fairly smooth.
2. Add rest of crust ingredients to food processor and blend until cookie dough consistency (generally forms a ball in the food processor).
3. Spread mixture in small, shallow tart pan or bowl. Press it down evenly and along sides of pan. If you do not have a tart pan available, you can form short walls on a plate and press the edges with fork to look like a pie crust.
4. Set in refrigerator to firm up while making tart filling.

Topping:

1. Blend all ingredients in the Topping list until smooth and creamy. Adjust measurements if needed and taste tartness level. Julie likes a very tart taste to balance the sweetness of the crust.
2. Remove crust from refrigerator.
3. Pour topping over crust so it fills the tart just below the rim.

4. Chill for a couple of hours in refrigerator. Serve cold so that the tart holds up and topping does not become runny. Garnish with a few lemon slices on the side.

JUICY MORSEL: Acidity and alkalinity are the hot topic lately. Have you heard people say, "I don't eat lemons; they are too acidic and I am trying to create an alkaline body?"

These folks are completely mistaken. Lemons are, in fact, acidic outside of the body. But as we eat them, they become alkaline due to their level of minerals and enzymes. Lemons are a raw foodist's staple and will not create high levels of acidity in the body.

People are becoming ridiculous when it comes to alkalinity obsession. Water manufacturers are trying to get us to buy alkaline water. Supplement manufacturers are selling alkalizing drops. This is overkill. The truth is that we need to eat a balance of dense greens and fresh fruits to keep alkaline. Nuts, seeds, grains, and dairy tend to be more acidic. You can still eat these foods and remain alkaline, but eat them in moderation. The bulk of your intake should be vegetables and fruit.

Do you think cavemen walked around with alkalinity drops to combat their acidic diet? Obviously not. So relax, and have a salad with some fresh lemon juice and follow it with a small slice of lemon tart.

MORE MOUSSE PLEASE! (Raw Vegan) by Julie

Serves 4

Ingredients:

½ cup raw cacao nibs

2 Tbsp. coconut butter (coconut oil is okay, butter is best)

¼ cup pine nuts

4 truly raw cashews

1/8 cup raw agave nectar

pinch sea salt

2 Tbsp. water (more if needed)

Toppings: seasonal fruit, or Julie's favorite, which includes ½ cup goji berries and 1 small carton of blueberries

Directions:

1. Blend cacao until as smooth and fine as possible (about 2-3 minutes). I recommend a food processor to keep the mousse chunky. If you blend with a high-powered blender such as Vita-Mix, your mousse will be much smoother. This recipe is for a thicker, chunkier mousse; almost as if it has chocolate chips in it.
2. Add other ingredients, minus the toppings, and blend again in food processor.
3. Spread onto center of plate, or in shallow bowl, leaving room around the edges to top with fruit later.

4. Chill at least one hour and serve with seasonal fruit or Julie's favorite: goji berries and blueberries. These should be nearly covering the mousse and all around the edges, so every bite of mousse has some fruit in it.
5. Drizzle a few cacao nibs over the top for decoration. Drizzle agave across the top for flare (optional). Julie loves flare. It makes her happy when she sees pretty designs of agave on a white plate with the gorgeous dessert in the middle!

JUICY MORSEL: Most of the pine nuts we purchase come from pine trees that are wild. We encourage you to look up pine nut harvesting and then get your own fresh ones! Why buy nuts that have been packaged and sat on a shelf for a year or so? Forage for your own the next time you hit the forest! (careful to check the correct pine types for harvest).

If we imagine ourselves harvesting pine nuts by hand (which is how it is still done), we know it is difficult to harvest more than a small handful at a time. This is generally a good amount to stick to when eating nuts. Eat about what you would be able to harvest, by hand, if you were foraging for food. This amount will prevent overdose on fats and acids that leads to indigestion.

PICK-YER-PUDDIN' (Raw Vegan) by Julie

Serves 1 adult or 2 children

Ingredients (for plain banana version):

½ red banana

¼ cup pine nuts

1 Tbsp. raw agave nectar

2 Tbsp. nut mylk (cashew is best)

pinch sea salt

Directions:

1. Blend all ingredients in food processor until smooth.
2. Variations on flavor are great for kids! Try blending in one of the following to the plain pudding and have them pick-their-puddin'! Let them choose from: ¼ cup strawberries, ½ tsp. cinnamon, ½ tsp. vanilla extract (or scrape inside of 1 vanilla bean), or 1 Tbsp. raw cacao powder.
3. Let chill in refrigerator for at least one hour for thick pudding consistency.

JUICY MORSEL: It can be a challenge to get children begging for raw food. We are always searching for things that Sarah's daughter, Ophena, will enjoy.

We have learned that giving her a sense of ownership in the food she is eating really helps. For example, we send her out to the garden to pick her plate of greens she must eat with dinner every evening.

When I first created the Pick-Yer-Puddin' recipe, I had Ophena do a taste test of the different flavors and give me feedback. Now she makes this dessert herself and adds her own flavors.

Sarah and I do not force Ophena to suddenly be a 100% raw food eater. We encourage her to try everything we make, eliminate all refined foods from the house, and involve her in recipe creations.

Ophena will often make up new recipes for The Healing Patch café we dream of opening. Perhaps you can give your children a project: "If you could open a raw food restaurant anywhere in the world, where would it be? What food would you serve? Write the recipes and create a menu. Draw a picture of the restaurant and then make me your favorite recipe!" The café ideas may take place in their imagination, but that is where most of their reality happens for them, anyway! Let them experiment and take ownership in a healthful lifestyle.

Ophena makes desktop art for us for our computers, with our business name. She is not something outside of our healthful lifestyle that we try to smuggle in; rather, she is an integral part of it.

SWEET STRAWBERRY PIE (Raw Vegan) by Sarah

Serves 2

Ingredients:

Crust:

1 date (with Julie, oops, I mean 1 date...like the fruit)
1 cup cashews
½ vanilla bean
1/3 tsp. cinnamon

Filling:

3 tsp. raw agave nectar
3 strawberries with greens attached
1 heaping Tbsp. raw honey

Topping:

2 strawberries
2 tsp. raw agave nectar
½ tsp. honey

Directions:

Crust:

1. PULSE all of the crust ingredients in a food processor, gently, until it starts to stick to the sides.

2. Add 1 Tbsp. water to mixture.
3. Blend until you get a ball of dough. If necessary, scrape the sides and blend again until a ball forms.
4. Use wax paper to press dough into a small bowl shape. The wax paper will keep the dough from sticking to your fingers. The crust bowl should be thick enough to form short walls, and sit up on its own, with no pan.

Filling:
1. Add all of the filling ingredients to food processor and PULSE a couple of times on low. Mixture should stay chunky like pie filling.
2. Put filling in a bowl and set aside.

Topping:
1. Add all of the topping ingredients to food processor.
2. Blend until you achieve a sauce consistency. This should be runnier than the filling.

Assembly:
1. Do not fill crust until ready to serve, as the fats tend to separate, and crust can turn white after a few minutes.
2. When ready to serve, pour filling into crust.
3. Drizzle the topping over the filling and over the crust. Some may be drizzled onto the plate as well.
4. Eat up and enjoy!

JUICY MORSEL: There is no need to throw away the green top of a strawberry. It generally tastes very mild and is full of extra minerals. We eat them in one big bite, with the strawberry itself, and can hardly taste them.

If you begin while your children are very young, and they do not know the difference, you can train them to enjoy the whole strawberry. So many kids eat one bite, and leave half of the strawberry still attached to the greens, because they are scared of eating the whole thing. Silly, silly. Enjoy the whole gift!

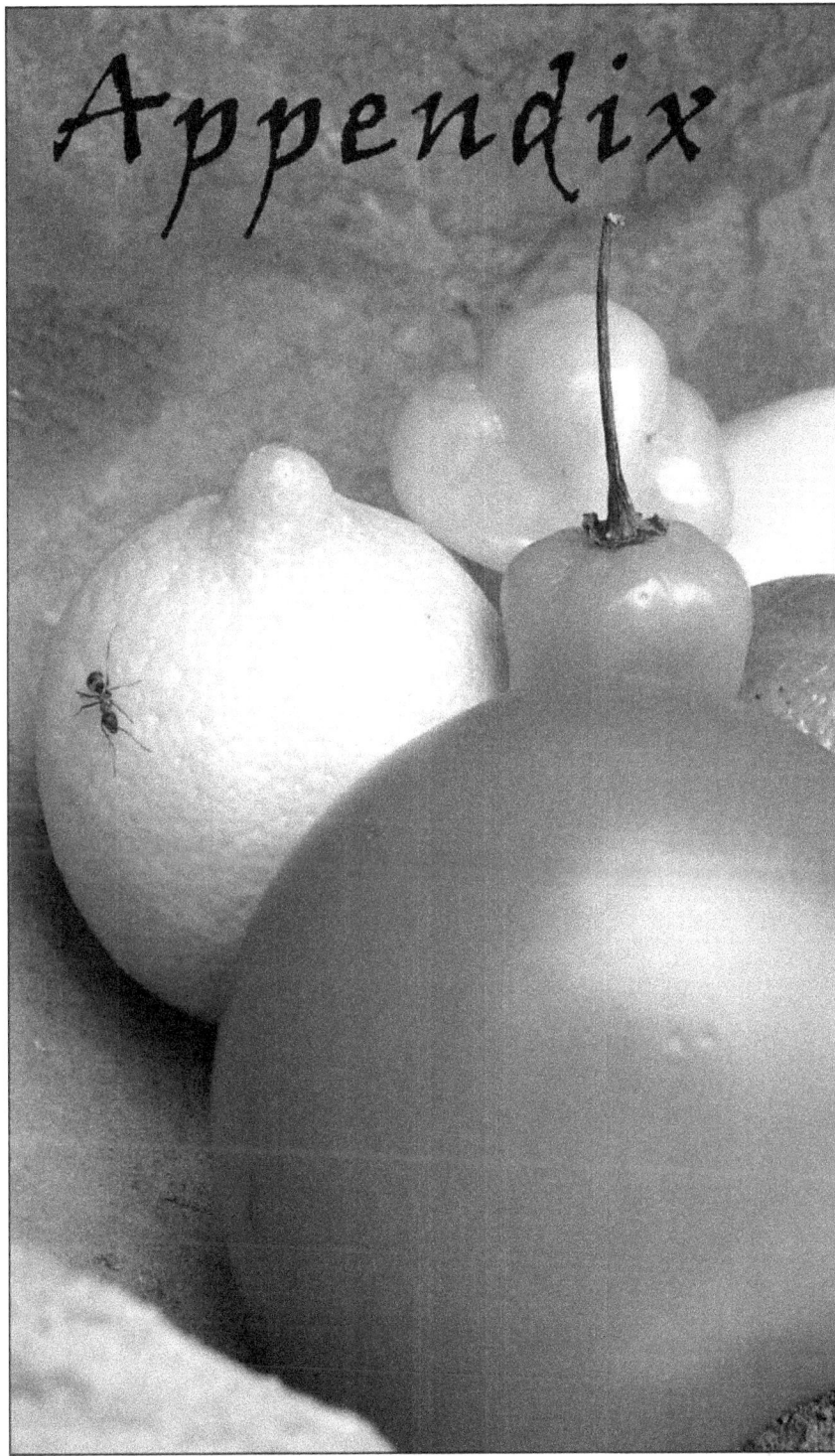
Appendix

THE "STAPLES"
(Also known as lifesavers to keep around at all times!)*

Agave Nectar

Bariani's Raw Organic Olive Oil

Bragg's Liquid Aminos

Bragg's Raw Apple Cider Vinegar

Cacao Nibs

Celtic Sea Salt

Dulse Flakes

Filtered water

Garlic cloves

Goji berries

Miso (do not purchase miso that sits on the shelf; use only miso that must be refrigerated at all times)

Nama Shoyu (raw, organic soy sauce)

Tahini

Truly Raw Cashews

Y.S. Organics Raw Honey

*Note: We do not think any, or all, of these items must be purchased to live a healthful raw food lifestyle. These items tend to be for people transitioning into vegetarian and raw foods. The list above provides more healthful options to mainstream condiments and cooking ingredients. One could very easily live a wonderful and fulfilling raw food lifestyle eating nothing but raw fruits and veggies straight from the plant! Many of the ingredients above are also expensive, initially, but you only need a small amount of them at a time. Everyone should choose what works best for them, but also be aware that this list is not written with the intention that raw foodists MUST drop a pretty penny for extras. We use these items as "accents" to predominantly whole food meals.

GLOSSARY

Agave Nectar: Agave is nectar derived from the agave plant, traditionally used to make tequila. The nectar is an alternative to sugary syrups, sugar cane, and other refined sweeteners that negatively effect blood sugar. It is low on the glycemic index and should be used in moderation for those looking to stabilize sweet cravings. Use only agave that says "raw." The darker ones are higher in mineral content. An even better choice is YACON syrup. It is even denser in nutrition, and lower on the glycemic index, but harder to find.

Blender (traditional): This blender is best for recipes that require gentle blending and chunkier textures, as opposed to smooth textures and complete blending. Any brand will do.

Cacao: This is chocolate in its raw state. Beans are the whole cacao form, nibs are the beans broken up into chunks, and powder is the bean pulverized into its finest form. No form is more healthful than the other; each is better suited to different recipes. Raw cacao is higher in antioxidants than ANY other food in the world! It is also loaded with magnesium, which helps with bone maintenance and stress levels.

Cashews (Truly Raw): Most raw cashews in the stores that say "raw" are not raw. They have been steam-opened. Some truly raw brands that are hand opened are Sunfood Nutrition and Navitas.

Coconut Butter vs. Coconut Oil: The butter is less greasy, as it is a mixture of coconut oil and the coconut meat. It also tends to be mildly sweet. The oil is the pure fat extracted from the coconut.

Dehydrator: A machine that eliminates the water from food, thereby preserving it, and creating a more crispy texture. Dehydrators may be used to make veggie chips, dried fruit, raw crackers, etc....

Goji Berries: Also known as wolf berries, these berries are readily available in dried form at health food stores. They are adaptogenic, meaning they help us adapt to stress and also help the body release human growth hormone. These berries are LOADED with antioxidants. Add them to everything you can!

Honey (Raw): Most honeys that claim to be raw are not, and contain a huge number of chemicals. The ABSOLUTE finest honey in quality and taste, we have found, is Y.S. Organics, sold in most health stores. There are others that are good, but we have not yet found better. If anyone knows of any, please feel free to send samples and information!

Probiotics: These are the beneficial bacteria that live throughout your body, many of which reside in the digestive tract. They are essential for the immune system and digestion. There are VERY few companies that naturally process their probiotics. The only ones I trust thus far are New Chapter, Garden of Life, and Megafood. There are other good ones, I am sure, but with these three brands you won't go wrong!

Raw: Raw refers to food that is heated to no higher than 118 degrees. This preserves enzymes, minerals, and vitamins. Raw food is essentially LIVE food that has all of the nutrition ready for dispersal in our bodies. While some raw foodists eat raw meat, we do not consider this to be a necessary, healthful, or planet-friendly choice and therefore do not use raw meat in any of our recipes. For more info on meat and the planet, a great source to read is <u>The Food Revolution</u> by John Robbins.

Salt: The only salt that should be used for our recipes is Celtic Sea Salt, Real Salt, or Himalayan crystal salt. Iodized salts should NEVER be used. They are toxic to the system and they are stripped of all natural and mineral benefit to the body. An excellent reference for salt information may be found in the book <u>Cleanse and Purify Thyself</u> by Richard Anderson.

Sprout Bag/Nut Mylk Bag: Found in most health food stores, these are the SAME thing: a netted bag that allows liquid to flow through and collects the solids. Can be used to sprout seeds, legumes, and grains, or to strain the mylk from the solids during nut milking (see our Nut Mylk recipe).

Vita-Mix: An extremely powerful blender that pulverizes the ingredients. Best for foods/beverages that need thorough mixing and smooth texture. BlendTec is another brand that will achieve the same result.

Young Coconut: Often called Thai coconut. They are higher in minerals than mature coconuts, have softer meat, and are full of tropical flavor! To open, use a chef's chopping knife and about 1-2 inches from center, use force to chop 4 even hits to the coconut in a circular shape. These 4 forceful chops should be enough to create a lid that can then be popped open (think of it like a pumpkin lid). There should be enough room to pour out the juice and then scoop out the meat, which is usually soft and slimy. If there is any purplish mold, bring it back for a refund, and get a fresh one!

SUGGESTED READING TO SUPPORT YOUR PHYSICAL AND SPIRITUAL HEALTH

Anastasia by Vladimir Megre

Cleanse and Purify Thyself by Richard Anderson

Eating for Beauty by David Wolfe

Excitotoxins: The Taste That Kills by Russell L. Blaylock

The Food Revolution by John Robbins

The Four Agreements: A Practical Guide to Personal Freedom (A Toltec Wisdom Book) by Don Miguel Ruiz

The Life Bridge by Paul Schulick, Thomas M. Newmark, and Richard Sarnat

LifeFood Recipe Book by Annie and David Jubb

The Secret Teachings of Plants: The Intelligence of the Heart in the Direct Perception of Nature by Stephen Harrod Buhner

The Sunfood Diet Success System by David Wolfe

Wild Fermentation by Sandor Ellix Katz

You Can Heal Your Life by Louise Hay

The 80/10/10 Diet by Dr. Douglas N. Graham

Full Name:

Sarah Michelle Woodward

Guilty Pleasure:

FOOD! I welcome all of it.

Worst Recipe ever made:

Egg dropping top ~~Ramen~~ Ramien (I was 11 years old)

Food you would walk to the moon for:

My mother's caper, fennel salmon. it's to die for!

Worst thing ever eaten:

Blue cheese stuffed olives or the meat in menudo

Inspiration/Instant Motivator:

Ophena's lectures (my daughter)

Favorite Kitchen Utensil:

The rice scraper (that I don't use for rice)

Reason for eating raw:

Um, let me think..... Cancer patient

Worst Kitchen manners:

tasting and tasting and tasting I'm usually not hungry by the time the

Favorite Family Recipe: meal is done

~~My mothers soups~~ oh wait, the Fennel, caper salmon!

Full Name: ♥ ♥ ♥ ♥ ♥ ♥

Julie Cara ~~Hoffenberg~~, lover of cheese

Guilty Pleasure:

Um, cheese! Aged cheddar, Brie, Feta, oh my!

Worst Recipe ever made:

I tried to make soup with leeks and every other veggie that was in my fridge. HORRIFIC! Utterly horrific.

Food you would walk to the moon for:

Once again, cheese. Need you ask? Thimbleberries & raspberries! Also, barakas, which Mom makes. They are a spinach & feta dish wrapped in dough (a traditional Greek recipe from my Great Grandmother)

Worst thing ever eaten:

Liver and shark (enter gagging sounds here)

Inspiration/Instant Motivator:

~~Coffee~~ (just kidding.) Laughing hysterically, the ocean, a hug, smells of nature, ... AAAHHH!

Favorite Kitchen Utensil:

My spatula (nothing makes for a happy gal like a bowl scraped completely clean of batter.)

Reason for eating raw:

I feel my healthiest & most vibrant on raw. Also, all the research shows no increase of lifeforce when cooking food.

Worst Kitchen manners:

I lick everything while cooking (even myself if something drips on me). I'm convinced saliva must make things taste better.

Favorite Family Recipe:

The Barakas mentioned above, Cream Cheese Spaghetti, Lox & Bagels, and everything my Grandma's ever made! (I like food. Yup.)

www.ingramcontent.com/pod-product-compliance
Lightning Source LLC
Chambersburg PA
CBHW071134280326
41935CB00010B/1228